This guide is made possible

by the support of Genentech BioOncology

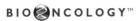

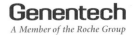

cure's Illustrated Guide to Cancer

SECOND EDITION

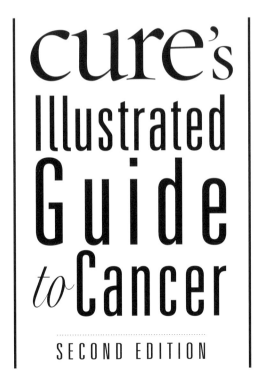

cure's Illustrated Guide to Cancer

SECOND EDITION

curemedia**group**

Dallas, Texas

Published by
CURE Media Group
3102 Oak Lawn Ave., Suite 610
Dallas, TX 75219
curetoday.com

Information presented is not intended as a substitute for the personalized professional advice given by a healthcare provider. The publishers urge readers to contact appropriately qualified health professionals for advice on any health or lifestyle change inspired by information herein.

This publication was produced by CURE Media Group through the financial support of Genentech. The views expressed in this publication are not necessarily those of Genentech or the publishers. Although great care has been taken to ensure accuracy, CURE Media Group and its servants or agents shall not be responsible or in any way liable for the continued currency of the information or for any errors, omissions or inaccuracies in this book, whether arising from negligence or otherwise or for any consequences arising therefrom. Parts of this book were first published in *CURE* magazine and are reprinted here in slightly different form. Review and creation of content is solely the responsibility of CURE Media Group. CURE Media Group is affiliated with McKesson Specialty Health, a division of McKesson Corporation.

Any mention of retail products does not constitute an endorsement by the authors or the publisher.

Library of Congress Control Number: 2012956178

ISBN 9780985911423

Editors: Lena Huang, Katherine Lagomarsino and Debu Tripathy, MD
Design: Susan Douglass
Layout: Glenn Zamora
Medical illustrations: Lewis E. Calver, Pam Curry, Erin Moore and Jim Perkins
Scientific advisor: Diane Gambill, PhD

Printed in the United States of America

Table *of* Contents

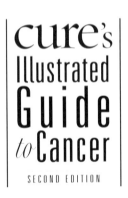

Introduction

We are pleased to present an update of *CURE's Illustrated Guide to Cancer*. In this second edition, we have included new diagrams and figures to accommodate the rapidly changing field of cancer diagnosis and treatment. This suite of illustrations has been carefully chosen from our extensive library. Our readers, which include patients, friends and family, physicians, nurses and other healthcare professionals, have cited our illustrations as the most helpful when it comes to explaining cancer. These pictorial descriptions provide a guided tour as to how different types of cancers are staged and greatly aid in the understanding of a diverse set of tumor types. The biological mechanisms that make cancer cells grow and spread are clearly summarized. Other diagrams give a sense of how various therapies work, including new targeted biological treatments. This knowledge can help patients participate in the decision-making process and give them a firm footing going forward.

We have extended the types of cancers covered, with less common cancers now included. New insights from the genomic revolution—a trend termed "personalized medicine," whereby cancer therapies are being tailored to individual tumor characteristics—are now reviewed in more detail. Innovations ranging from organ-preserving surgical techniques to stem cell transplantation are depicted with a clarity readers have come to expect from *CURE* magazine. *CURE's Illustrated Guide to Cancer Second Edition* is an atlas, a map, a storybook—designed to empower you in the best way—with knowledge.

Debu Tripathy, MD

Editor-in-Chief, *CURE* Magazine

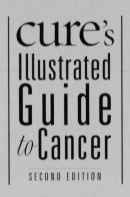

Chapter 1

About Cancer

CANCER ORIGINATES from the uncontrolled growth of abnormal cells. In the body, normal cells follow a pattern of growth, division and death. However, cancer cells follow their own pattern—growing, dividing and forming more abnormal cells. This growth may occur in adjacent cells, or cancerous cells may travel to distant locations in the body through the blood or lymphatic system, which is called metastasis. There are many types of cancer, and cancer cells can develop in different parts of the body. Some cancer cells form solid tumors while others involve the blood or bone marrow. Cancer strikes people of all ages, although the risk of many cancers increases with age.

Tumor Environment

The complex environment in which a tumor thrives plays a role in cancer growth and metastasis.

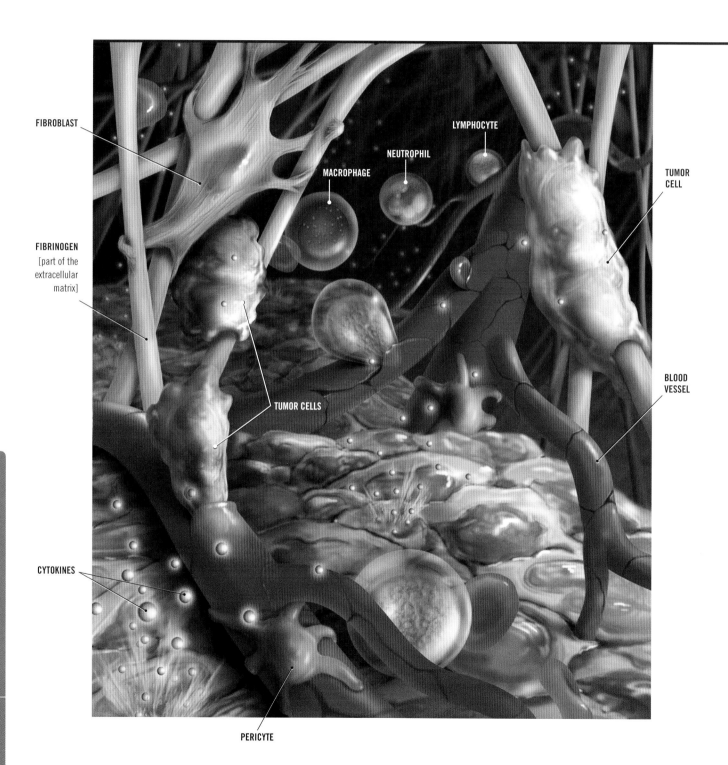

FIBROBLAST

FIBRINOGEN
[part of the
extracellular
matrix]

MACROPHAGE

NEUTROPHIL

LYMPHOCYTE

TUMOR
CELL

TUMOR CELLS

BLOOD
VESSEL

CYTOKINES

PERICYTE

ELEMENTS IN THE TUMOR ENVIRONMENT >

BLOOD VESSELS that nourish the tumor are "leaky" and have other differences compared with normal blood vessels. They are, therefore, the target of some current cancer-fighting drugs in a class known as antiangiogenics.

CYTOKINES, immune system–signaling molecules that contribute to inflammation, can promote tumor blood vessel growth, sustain viability of dangerous precancerous cells and prompt some cells to reproduce faster, increasing their risk of mutation.

NEUTROPHILS and **LYMPHOCYTES** are immune system cells that can tip the balance toward a cancer-promoting or cancer-inhibiting microenvironment. An abundance of neutrophils is associated with increased growth of tumor blood vessels and a poor prognosis. High levels of lymphocytes have been linked to a better prognosis.

FIBRINOGEN, which normally plays a role in clot formation, may indirectly affect tumor growth, metastasis and blood vessel formation.

TUMOR CELLS, cancer-associated **FIBROBLASTS,** immune system components known as tumor-associated **MACROPHAGES** and **PERICYTES,** which are cells adjacent to the tumor blood vessel lining, release enzymes that alter the structure of the extracellular matrix. Remodeling the matrix—the scaffolding of tissue that supports cells—makes it easier for tumors to invade and spread.

ILLUSTRATION BY PAM CURRY
ORIGINALLY PUBLISHED IN "BAD NEIGHBORS," *CURE* WINTER 2009

Metastasis

Cancer cells may travel to distant parts of the body through the blood or lymphatic system, which is called metastasis.

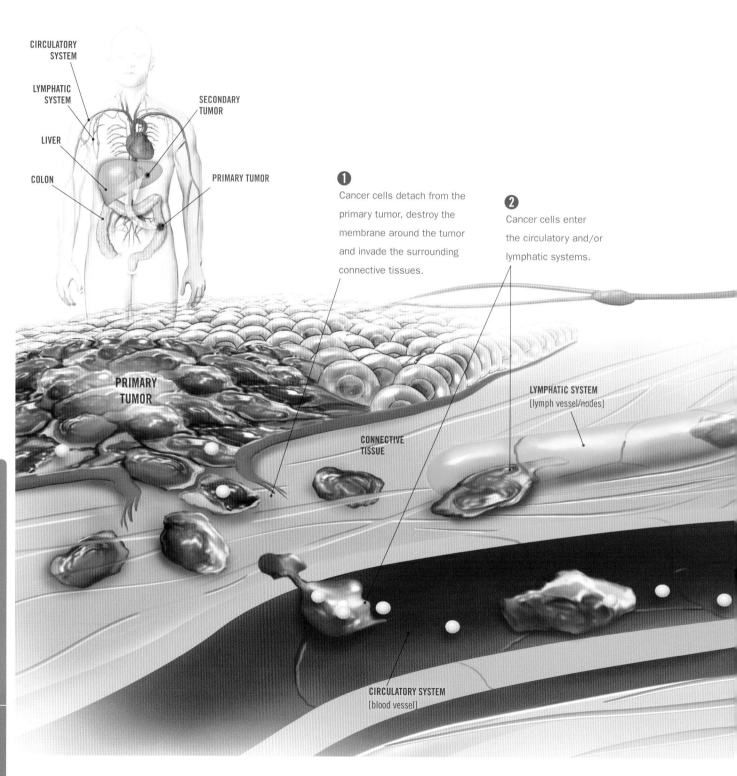

CIRCULATORY SYSTEM

LYMPHATIC SYSTEM

LIVER

COLON

SECONDARY TUMOR

PRIMARY TUMOR

1 Cancer cells detach from the primary tumor, destroy the membrane around the tumor and invade the surrounding connective tissues.

2 Cancer cells enter the circulatory and/or lymphatic systems.

PRIMARY TUMOR

CONNECTIVE TISSUE

LYMPHATIC SYSTEM
[lymph vessel/nodes]

CIRCULATORY SYSTEM
[blood vessel]

ABOUT CANCER

1

How *does* Cancer Metastasize?

WHEN CANCER CELLS SPREAD to one or more sites in the body, they often travel through the **lymph system** or the **bloodstream**. Only a few cells will survive every stage of development, but a few are all it takes for metastasis to occur. Regardless of whether the metastasis is regional (in the lymph nodes, tissues or organs close to the primary site) or distant (in organs or tissues that are farther away), it is always named for the place it began. **That's why colon cancer that spreads to the liver is called metastatic colorectal cancer, not liver cancer.**

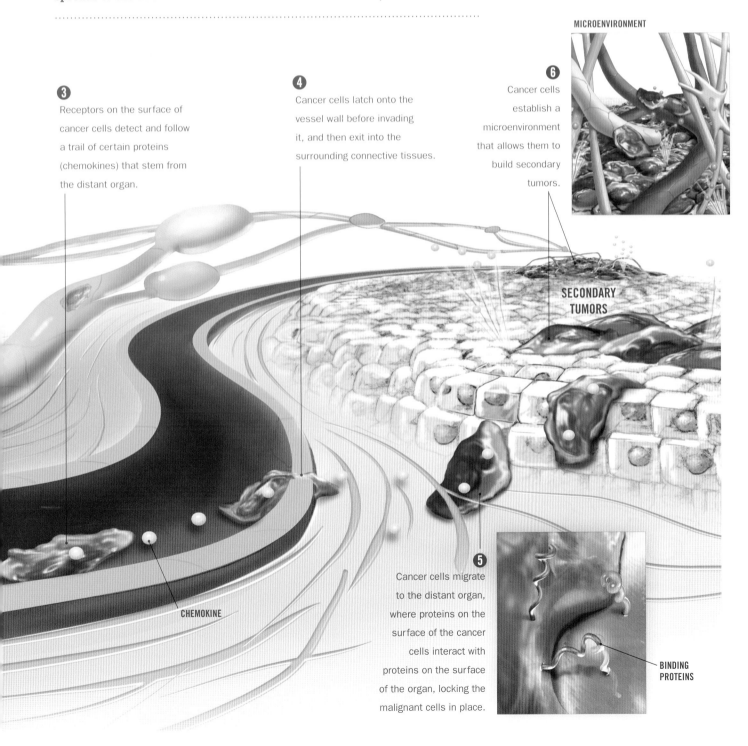

MICROENVIRONMENT

❸
Receptors on the surface of cancer cells detect and follow a trail of certain proteins (chemokines) that stem from the distant organ.

❹
Cancer cells latch onto the vessel wall before invading it, and then exit into the surrounding connective tissues.

❻
Cancer cells establish a microenvironment that allows them to build secondary tumors.

SECONDARY TUMORS

CHEMOKINE

❺
Cancer cells migrate to the distant organ, where proteins on the surface of the cancer cells interact with proteins on the surface of the organ, locking the malignant cells in place.

BINDING PROTEINS

ILLUSTRATION BY PAM CURRY
ORIGINALLY PUBLISHED IN "GUESSING GAME," *SPECIAL REPORT ON METASTATIC CANCER, CURE* SUPPLEMENT 2012

Cause and Effect

[Cancer can be caused by environmental factors, random events or hereditary factors.]

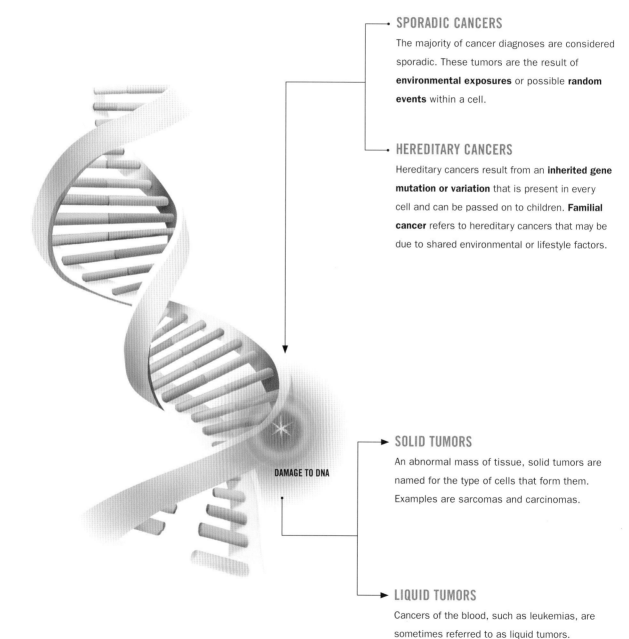

SPORADIC CANCERS

The majority of cancer diagnoses are considered sporadic. These tumors are the result of **environmental exposures** or possible **random events** within a cell.

HEREDITARY CANCERS

Hereditary cancers result from an **inherited gene mutation or variation** that is present in every cell and can be passed on to children. **Familial cancer** refers to hereditary cancers that may be due to shared environmental or lifestyle factors.

DAMAGE TO DNA

SOLID TUMORS

An abnormal mass of tissue, solid tumors are named for the type of cells that form them. Examples are sarcomas and carcinomas.

LIQUID TUMORS

Cancers of the blood, such as leukemias, are sometimes referred to as liquid tumors.

ABOUT CANCER

1

ILLUSTRATION BY PAM CURRY
ORIGINALLY PUBLISHED IN "WHAT IS CANCER?" *CURE'S 2007 CANCER RESOURCE GUIDE*

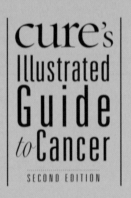

cure's Illustrated Guide to Cancer

SECOND EDITION

Chapter 2

Cancer Staging

STAGING, an integral part of the cancer diagnosis, helps physicians determine the patient's treatment plan and prognosis. It also provides nurses, healthcare providers, doctors and researchers a common language to discuss a patient's cancer. Staging describes the extent of the cancer. For most cancers, it is based on location of the primary tumor, size of the tumor, number of tumors present and whether the cancer has spread to nearby organs, tissues, lymph nodes or distant parts of the body. TNM staging is the most commonly used system and is based on T, the primary tumor or place where the cancer began; N, the level of lymph node involvement; and M, the presence or absence of metastasis.

Cancer Staging

Staging defines how much cancer exists and whether the cancer has spread to other parts of the body. General staging information varies for specific kinds of cancer.

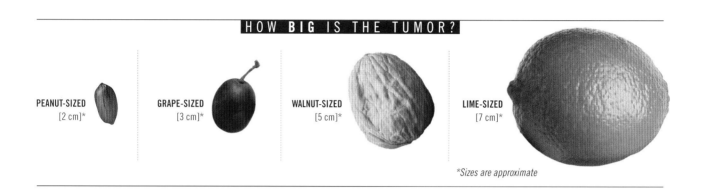

HOW **BIG** IS THE TUMOR?

PEANUT-SIZED
[2 cm]*

GRAPE-SIZED
[3 cm]*

WALNUT-SIZED
[5 cm]*

LIME-SIZED
[7 cm]*

*Sizes are approximate

Typical TNM Tumor Staging System

Primary Tumor (T)	
TX	Primary tumor cannot be evaluated
T0	No evidence of primary tumor
Tis	Carcinoma in situ (non-invasive)
T1, T2, T3, T4	Depends on size and/or extent of primary tumor
Regional Lymph Nodes (N)	
NX	Regional lymph nodes cannot be evaluated
N0	No regional lymph node involvement
N1, N2, N3	Depends on number and location of spread to regional lymph nodes
Distant Metastasis (M)	
MX	Distant metastasis cannot be evaluated
M0	Cancer has not spread to other parts of the body
M1	Cancer has spread to other parts of the body

Overall Stage Groupings

STAGE	DESCRIPTION
Stage 0	Carcinoma in situ (non-invasive)
Stage 1 to 3	More extensive disease indicated by higher numbers (could include larger tumor, cancer present in nearby lymph nodes and/or cancer present in organs adjacent to the organ in which the cancer began)
Stage 4	Cancer has spread to a distant organ (metastasized)

CANCER STAGING

2

ORIGINALLY PUBLISHED IN "PATHOLOGY & STAGING," *CURE'S 2007 CANCER RESOURCE GUIDE*

Noninvasive Breast Cancer

[Each cellular change of noninvasive breast cancer involves various screening and management recommendations.]

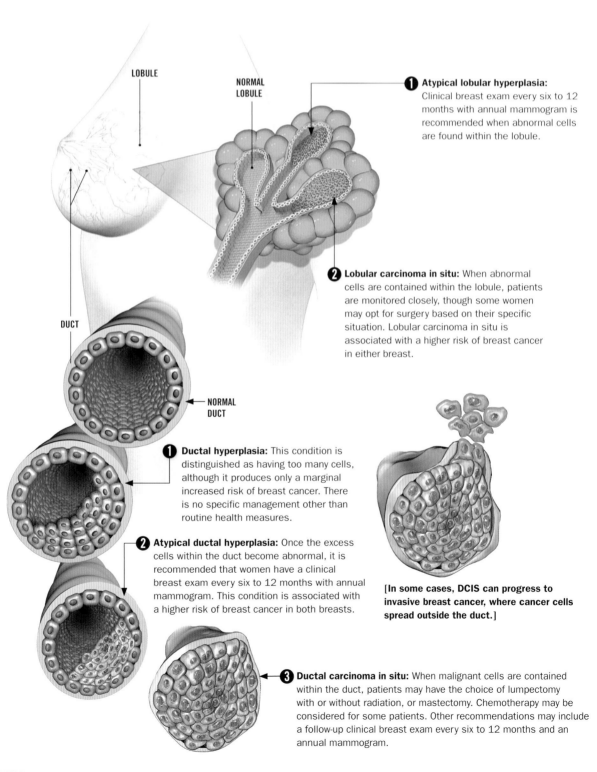

LOBULE

NORMAL LOBULE

❶ Atypical lobular hyperplasia: Clinical breast exam every six to 12 months with annual mammogram is recommended when abnormal cells are found within the lobule.

❷ Lobular carcinoma in situ: When abnormal cells are contained within the lobule, patients are monitored closely, though some women may opt for surgery based on their specific situation. Lobular carcinoma in situ is associated with a higher risk of breast cancer in either breast.

DUCT

NORMAL DUCT

❶ Ductal hyperplasia: This condition is distinguished as having too many cells, although it produces only a marginal increased risk of breast cancer. There is no specific management other than routine health measures.

❷ Atypical ductal hyperplasia: Once the excess cells within the duct become abnormal, it is recommended that women have a clinical breast exam every six to 12 months with annual mammogram. This condition is associated with a higher risk of breast cancer in both breasts.

[In some cases, DCIS can progress to invasive breast cancer, where cancer cells spread outside the duct.]

❸ Ductal carcinoma in situ: When malignant cells are contained within the duct, patients may have the choice of lumpectomy with or without radiation, or mastectomy. Chemotherapy may be considered for some patients. Other recommendations may include a follow-up clinical breast exam every six to 12 months and an annual mammogram.

ILLUSTRATION BY ERIN MOORE
ORIGINALLY PUBLISHED IN "IS IT REALLY CANCER?" *CURE* FALL 2006
SOURCE: *ANNALS OF INTERNAL MEDICINE*; *CURE* RESEARCH

Invasive Breast Cancer

[
The American Joint Committee on Cancer's TNM staging system is the standard system used to classify breast cancer.
]

The TNM staging system is based on T, for tumor; N, for spread to the lymph nodes; and M, for metastasis (spread to distant tissues or organs). Additional letters or numbers, which provide more details of the tumor, lymph nodes or metastasis, may follow the TNM stages.

STAGE T:

TØ: No evidence of primary tumor.

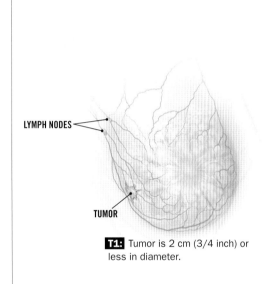

LYMPH NODES

TUMOR

T1: Tumor is 2 cm (3/4 inch) or less in diameter.

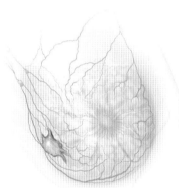

T2: Tumor is more than 2 cm but less than 5 cm (2 inches) in diameter.

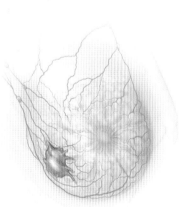

T3: Tumor is more than 5 cm in diameter.

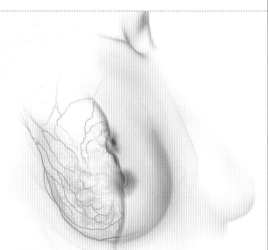

T4: Tumor is any size and has grown into the chest wall or skin, or has been diagnosed as inflammatory breast cancer.

2

N0: Cancer has not spread to nearby lymph nodes.

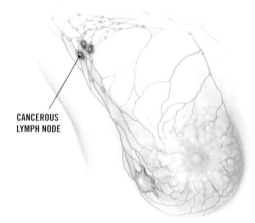

CANCEROUS
LYMPH NODE

N1: Cancer has spread to 1 to 3 underarm lymph nodes and/or to the internal mammary lymph nodes found by sentinel lymph node biopsy.

STAGE M:

M0: No spread to distant tissues or organs is found on imaging procedures or by physical exam.

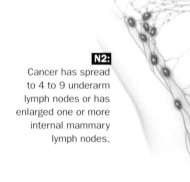

N2: Cancer has spread to 4 to 9 underarm lymph nodes or has enlarged one or more internal mammary lymph nodes.

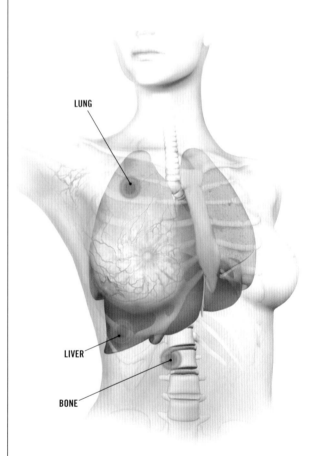

LUNG

LIVER

BONE

M1: The cancer has spread to distant tissues or organs, with the most common sites being bone, lung, brain and liver.

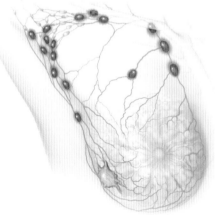

N3: Described as one of the following:

■ Cancer has spread to 10 or more underarm lymph nodes with at least one area measuring more than 2 mm. (N3a)

■ Cancer has spread to the lymph nodes under the collarbone with at least one area measuring more than 2 mm. (N3a)

■ Cancer has spread to one or more underarm lymph nodes with at least one area measuring more than 2 mm, and has enlarged one or more internal mammary lymph nodes. (N3b)

■ Cancer has spread to four or more underarm lymph nodes with

at least one area measuring more than 2 mm, and to the internal mammary lymph nodes found by sentinel lymph node biopsy. (N3b)

■ Cancer has spread to the lymph nodes above the collarbone with at least one area measuring more than 2 mm. (N3c)

Prostate Cancer

When diagnosing prostate cancer, doctors consider staging and grading. In grading, a score is assigned based on the Gleason grading system.

STAGE 1:

The cancer is located on one side of the prostate. At this stage, the tumor is very small or found incidentally, possibly during surgery or by an elevated prostate-specific antigen (PSA) level. The Gleason score is low.

STAGE 2:

The cancer is located only in the prostate but can be seen on imaging scans or felt during a digital rectal exam. The Gleason score may range from 2 to 10.

CANCER STAGING

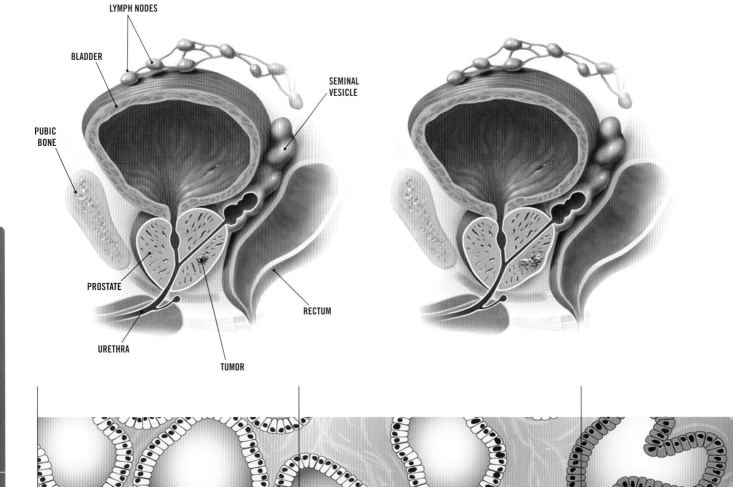

LYMPH NODES

BLADDER

SEMINAL VESICLE

PUBIC BONE

PROSTATE

RECTUM

URETHRA

TUMOR

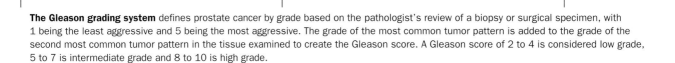

GRADE 1　　　GRADE 2　　　GRADE 3

The Gleason grading system defines prostate cancer by grade based on the pathologist's review of a biopsy or surgical specimen, with 1 being the least aggressive and 5 being the most aggressive. The grade of the most common tumor pattern is added to the grade of the second most common tumor pattern in the tissue examined to create the Gleason score. A Gleason score of 2 to 4 is considered low grade, 5 to 7 is intermediate grade and 8 to 10 is high grade.

STAGE 3:

The cancer has extended through the outer layer of the prostate and into surrounding tissues and may be found in the seminal vesicle but not in the lymph nodes. The Gleason score may range from 2 to 10.

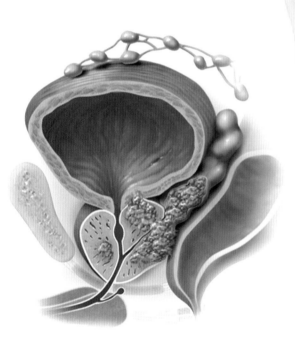

STAGE 4:

The cancer has spread to the lymph nodes near or far from the prostate or has spread to distant tissues or organs, such as the liver or bones. The Gleason score may range from 2 to 10.

CANCEROUS LYMPH NODES

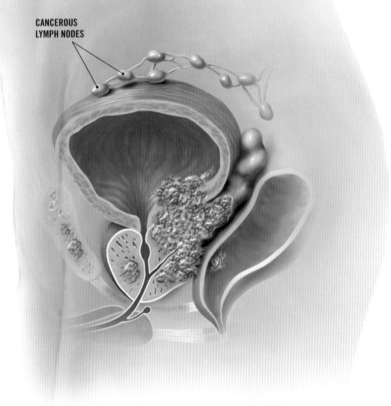

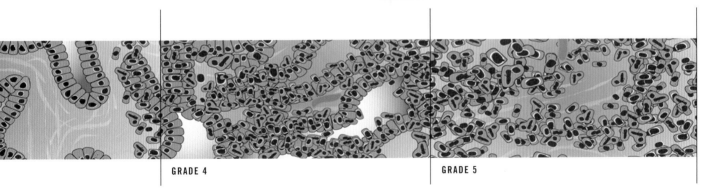

GRADE 4

GRADE 5

ILLUSTRATION BY PAM CURRY
ORIGINALLY PUBLISHED IN *CURE'S ILLUSTRATED GUIDE TO CANCER*, 2010

Non-Small Cell Lung Cancer

Following a lung cancer diagnosis, staging determines the best options for treatment. Many factors are evaluated, including the size of the tumor and the extent of spread.

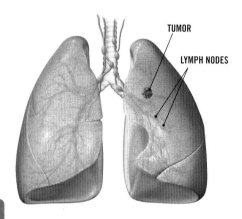

TUMOR

LYMPH NODES

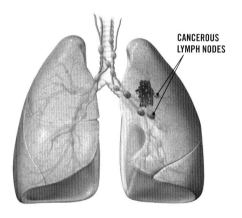

CANCEROUS LYMPH NODES

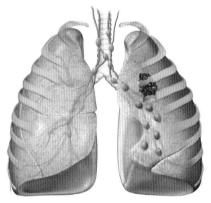

STAGE 1: The cancer is small (no larger than 3 cm for stage 1A; up to 5 cm for stage 1B) and has not spread to the lymph nodes.

STAGE 2: The tumor is up to 7 cm in diameter and may have spread to nearby lymph nodes.

STAGE 3A: The cancer has started to extend into surrounding tissues and structures, such as the lining of the lung and chest wall, and has spread to lymph nodes on the same side of the chest as the tumor.

TREATMENT OPTIONS:

SURGERY

ADJUVANT CHEMOTHERAPY

RADIATION THERAPY & CHEMOTHERAPY

CANCER STAGING

2

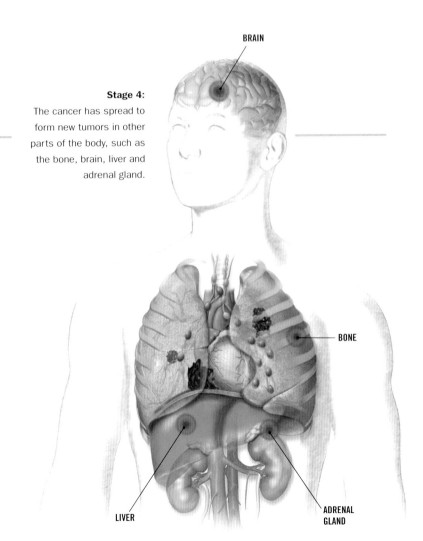

BRAIN

Stage 4:
The cancer has spread to form new tumors in other parts of the body, such as the bone, brain, liver and adrenal gland.

BONE

LIVER

ADRENAL GLAND

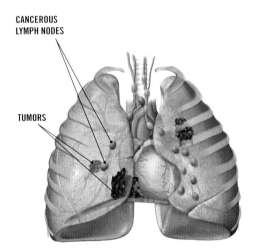

CANCEROUS LYMPH NODES

TUMORS

STAGE 3B: Two or more tumors are present, and the cancer has spread to the lung and lymph nodes on the opposite side of the chest.

ILLUSTRATION BY ERIN MOORE
ORIGINALLY PUBLISHED IN "LUNG OVERDUE," *CURE* SPRING 2010

Colon Cancer

There are several systems to stage colon cancer, but the most commonly used system was developed by the American Joint Committee on Cancer.

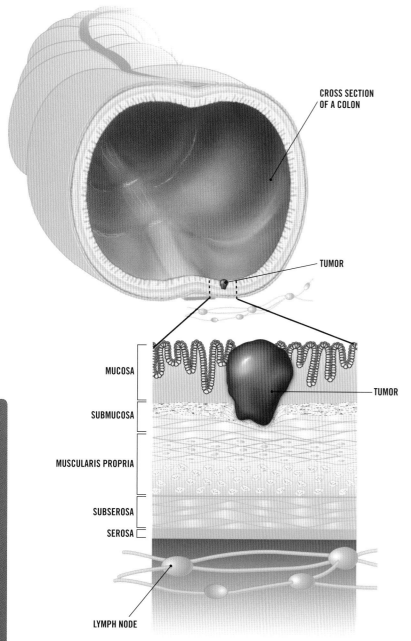

CROSS SECTION OF A COLON

TUMOR

MUCOSA

TUMOR

SUBMUCOSA

MUSCULARIS PROPRIA

SUBSEROSA

SEROSA

LYMPH NODE

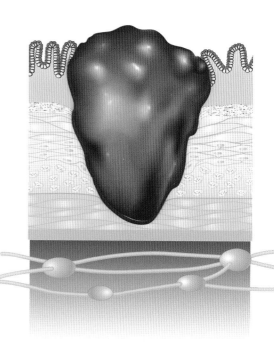

STAGE 1: The cancer has grown through the mucosa, or inner layer of the colon, and extends to the submucosa.

STAGE 2: The cancer has grown through the submucosa and into the next layer, the muscularis propria. It may or may not extend into the next layers, the subserosa or serosa, or to nearby tissues or organs. It has not spread to the lymph nodes.

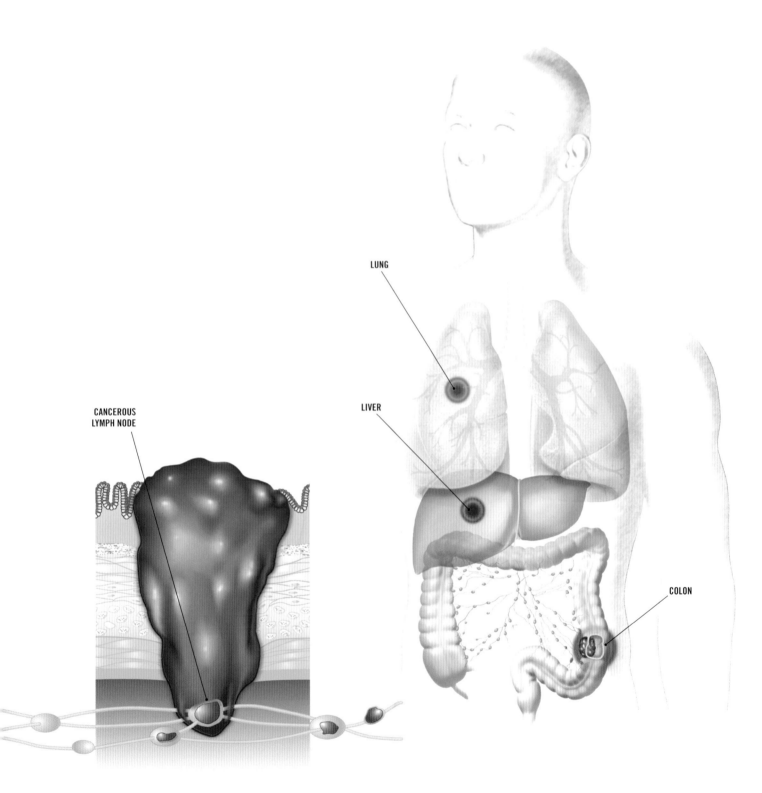

CANCEROUS LYMPH NODE

LUNG

LIVER

COLON

STAGE 3: The cancer may or may not have grown through the wall of the colon, but it has spread to nearby lymph nodes. It has not spread to distant tissues or organs.

STAGE 4: The cancer has spread to distant sites, such as the liver or lung. It may or may not have grown through the wall of the colon. It may or may not have spread to nearby lymph nodes.

ILLUSTRATION BY ERIN MOORE
ORIGINALLY PUBLISHED IN *CURE'S ILLUSTRATED GUIDE TO CANCER*, 2010

Chronic Lymphocytic Leukemia

The Rai staging system is typically used to describe chronic lymphocytic leukemia, a cancer of the blood.

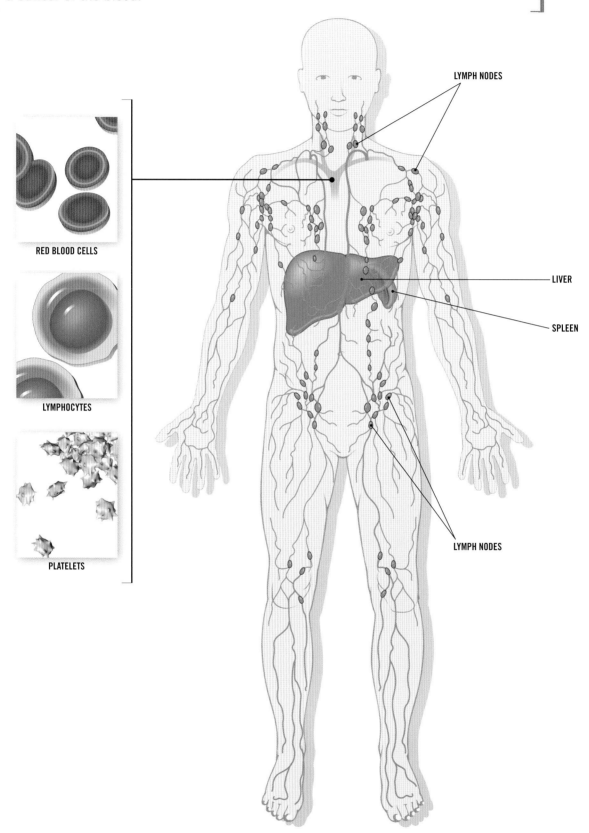

RED BLOOD CELLS

LYMPHOCYTES

PLATELETS

LYMPH NODES

LIVER

SPLEEN

LYMPH NODES

The Rai staging system includes five stages:

STAGE 0:

A high number of lymphocytes, a type of white blood cell, are found in the blood, a condition called lymphocytosis (a lymphocyte count greater than 15,000 cells per cubic millimeter). In this stage, the lymph nodes, spleen and liver are not enlarged. Red blood cell and platelet counts are in normal range.

STAGE 1:

In addition to lymphocytosis, the lymph nodes are swollen. The spleen and liver are not enlarged. Red blood cell and platelet counts are in normal range.

STAGE 2:

In addition to lymphocytosis, the spleen and/or liver are enlarged. The lymph nodes may or may not be swollen. Red blood cell and platelet counts are in normal range.

STAGE 3:

In addition to lymphocytosis, red blood cell counts are low, a condition called anemia. The spleen and/or liver may or may not be enlarged. The lymph nodes may or may not be swollen. Platelet counts are in normal range.

STAGE 4:

In addition to lymphocytosis, platelet counts are low, a condition called thrombocytopenia. The spleen and/or liver may or may not be enlarged. The lymph nodes may or may not be swollen. Red blood cell counts may or may not be low.

In addition, healthcare providers may divide these stages into risk groups when discussing treatment options. Stage 0 is regarded as low risk. Stages 1 and 2 are regarded as intermediate risk. Stages 3 and 4 are regarded as high risk.

ILLUSTRATION BY JIM PERKINS
ORIGINALLY PUBLISHED IN *CURE'S ILLUSTRATED GUIDE TO CANCER*, 2010

Hodgkin Lymphoma

The Ann Arbor staging system is used to describe the stages of Hodgkin lymphoma in adults. The same system can be used for non-Hodgkin lymphoma.

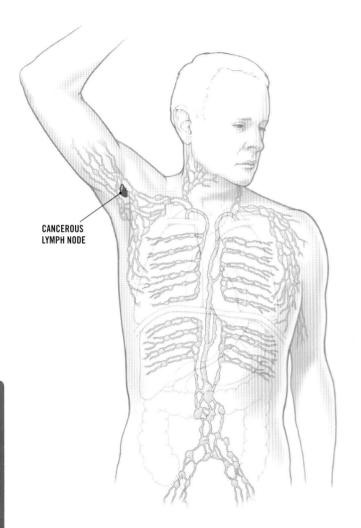

CANCEROUS
LYMPH NODE

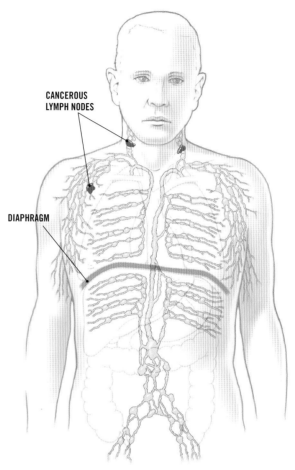

CANCEROUS
LYMPH NODES

DIAPHRAGM

STAGE 1:
The cancer is located in a lymph node or nodes in a single lymph node group.

STAGE 1E:
The cancer is located in one organ or in one area outside the lymph nodes (extranodal).

STAGE 2:
The cancer is located in two or more lymph node groups on the same side of the diaphragm.

STAGE 2E:
The cancer is located in one or more lymph node groups on the same side of the diaphragm and in an organ or area outside the lymph nodes.

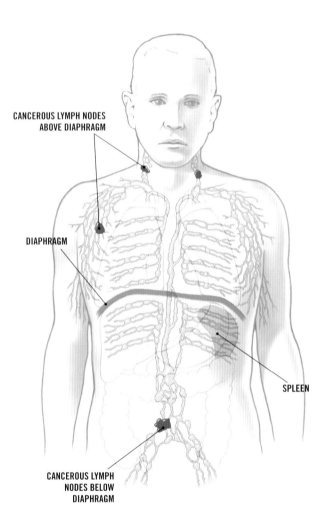

CANCEROUS LYMPH NODES ABOVE DIAPHRAGM

DIAPHRAGM

SPLEEN

CANCEROUS LYMPH NODES BELOW DIAPHRAGM

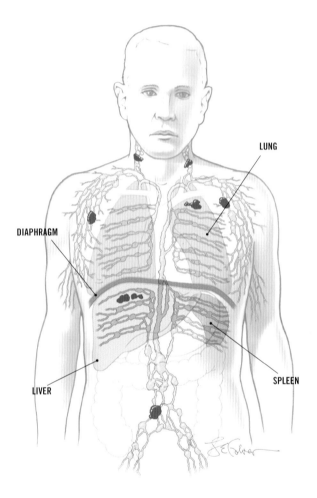

LUNG

DIAPHRAGM

LIVER

SPLEEN

STAGE 3: The cancer is located in one or more lymph node groups above and below the diaphragm.

STAGE 3E: The cancer is located in lymph node groups above and below the diaphragm and in an organ or area outside the lymph nodes.

STAGE 3S: The cancer is located in lymph node groups above and below the diaphragm and in the spleen.

STAGE 3S+E: The cancer is located in lymph node groups above and below the diaphragm, in the spleen and in an organ or area outside the lymph nodes.

STAGE 4: The cancer has spread outside the lymph nodes to one or more distant organs, such as the liver, lung or bone marrow.

Melanoma

Experts have outlined the following staging system to define the development of melanoma and determine the treatment course.

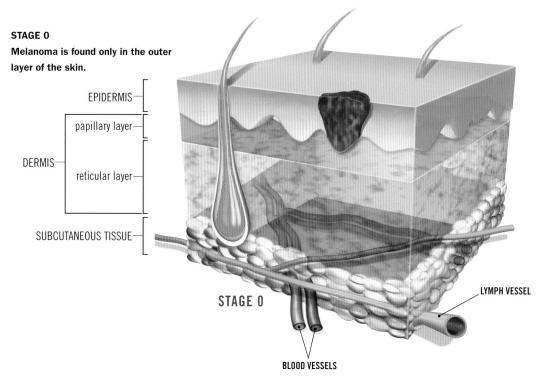

STAGE 0

Melanoma is found only in the outer layer of the skin.

EPIDERMIS

papillary layer

DERMIS

reticular layer

SUBCUTANEOUS TISSUE

STAGE 0

LYMPH VESSEL

BLOOD VESSELS

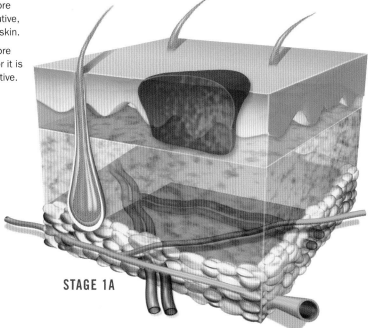

STAGE 1

Divided into two stages:

[Stage 1A] – The tumor is not more than 1 mm thick and is not ulcerative, meaning there is no break in the skin.

[Stage 1B] – The tumor is not more than 1 mm thick and ulcerative, or it is 1 to 2 mm thick and is not ulcerative.

STAGE 1A

CANCER STAGING

2

STAGE 2

Divided into three stages:

[Stage 2A] – The tumor is 1 to 2 mm thick with ulceration, or 2 to 4 mm thick with no ulceration.

[Stage 2B] – The tumor is 2 to 4 mm thick with ulceration, or more than 4 mm thick with no ulceration.

[Stage 2C] – The tumor is more than 4 mm thick and ulcerative.

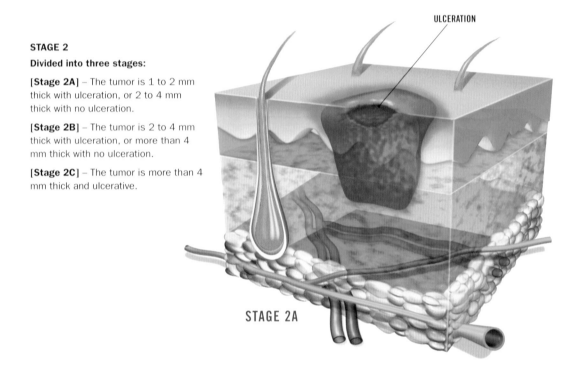

ULCERATION

STAGE 2A

STAGE 3

The tumor may be of any thickness, with or without ulceration, and has spread to one or more nearby lymph nodes; divided into three stages:

[Stage 3A] – The tumor may have spread to as many as three lymph nodes, but the tumor in the lymph node can only be seen under a microscope.

[Stage 3B] – The tumor has spread to as many as three lymph nodes, or the melanoma has not spread to the lymph nodes but has produced satellite tumors.

[Stage 3C] – The tumor has spread to four or more lymph nodes or has clinically evident positive lymph nodes.

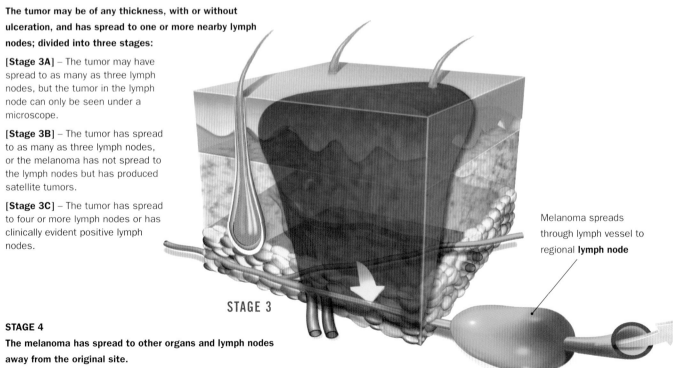

Melanoma spreads through lymph vessel to regional **lymph node**

STAGE 3

STAGE 4

The melanoma has spread to other organs and lymph nodes away from the original site.

ILLUSTRATION BY ERIN MOORE
ORIGINALLY PUBLISHED IN "ONLY SKIN DEEP," *CURE* SPRING 2003

Bladder Cancer

[Depending on the stage, bladder cancer may be treated with a simple surgical procedure, radiation, chemotherapy, removal of the bladder or a combination of these treatments.]

STAGE 2 OR 3:
Tumor has invaded the muscle wall or has reached beyond the muscle layer into the fatty tissues and may have spread to the reproductive organs. Surgical treatment is usually a radical cystectomy (removal of the bladder as well as other structures, including the uterus in women and the prostate in men). Urine is collected from the kidneys in an internal reservoir and emptied through the urethra or abdominal wall. In some cases, a partial cystectomy (removing the part of the bladder with cancer) or a simple cystectomy (removing the bladder only) might be possible. Surgery is often followed by radiation and/or chemotherapy.

STAGE 4:
Tumor has grown through the bladder wall and into the abdomen or pelvis. It may also have spread to nearby lymph nodes or distant sites, such as bones, liver or lungs. Treatment includes **chemotherapy with or without radiation therapy.** Surgery (cystectomy) might follow chemotherapy in some patients.

STAGE 1:
Tumor has formed in the lining of the bladder and may have invaded the connective tissue. A simple surgical procedure, **transurethral resection of the bladder tumor (TURBT),** may be used to remove the cancer.

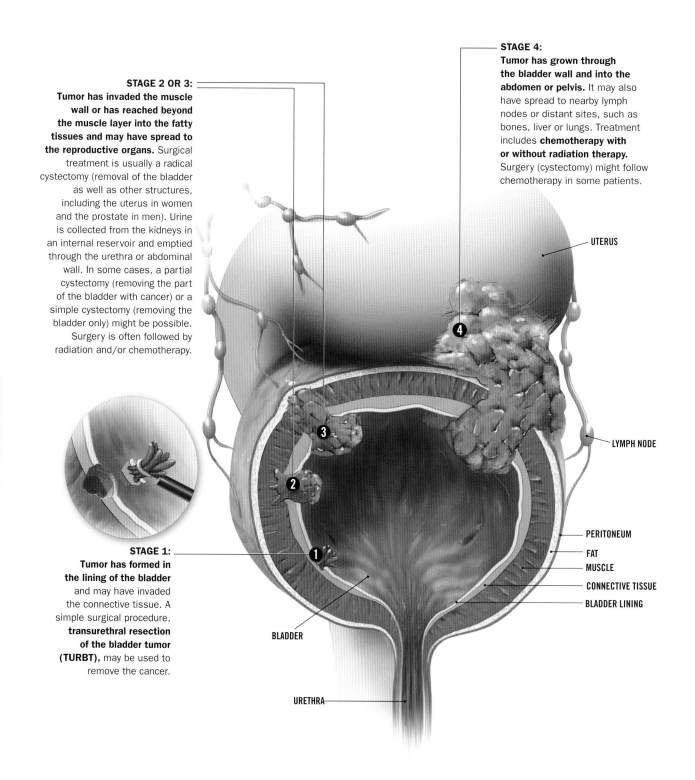

UTERUS

LYMPH NODE

PERITONEUM

FAT

MUSCLE

CONNECTIVE TISSUE

BLADDER LINING

BLADDER

URETHRA

ILLUSTRATION BY PAM CURRY
ORIGINALLY PUBLISHED IN "GOING THE DISTANCE," *CURE* SPRING 2012

Multiple Myeloma

[Multiple myeloma begins with a single precancerous plasma cell that multiplies uncontrollably and can eventually cause bone lesions and anemia.]

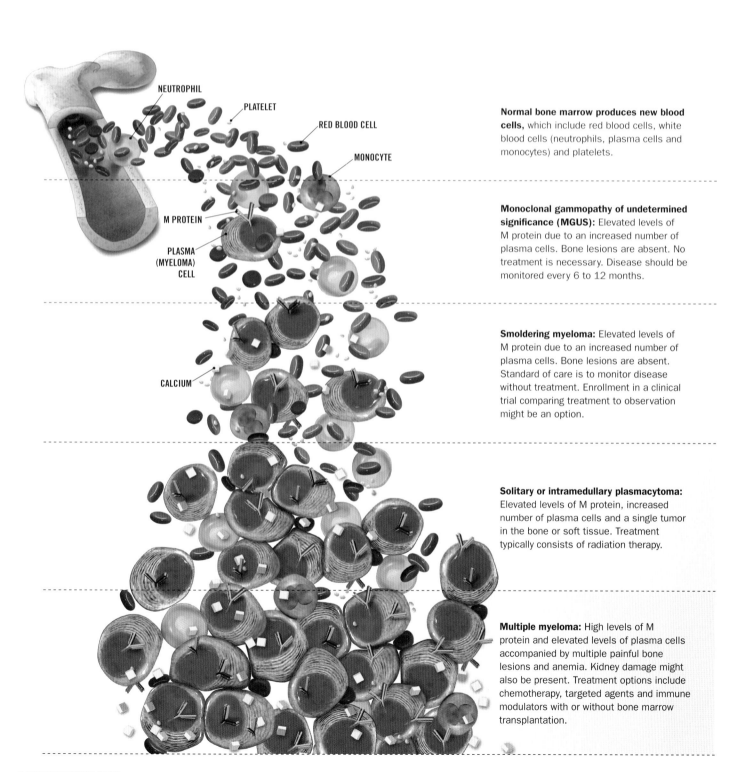

Normal bone marrow produces new blood cells, which include red blood cells, white blood cells (neutrophils, plasma cells and monocytes) and platelets.

Monoclonal gammopathy of undetermined significance (MGUS): Elevated levels of M protein due to an increased number of plasma cells. Bone lesions are absent. No treatment is necessary. Disease should be monitored every 6 to 12 months.

Smoldering myeloma: Elevated levels of M protein due to an increased number of plasma cells. Bone lesions are absent. Standard of care is to monitor disease without treatment. Enrollment in a clinical trial comparing treatment to observation might be an option.

Solitary or intramedullary plasmacytoma: Elevated levels of M protein, increased number of plasma cells and a single tumor in the bone or soft tissue. Treatment typically consists of radiation therapy.

Multiple myeloma: High levels of M protein and elevated levels of plasma cells accompanied by multiple painful bone lesions and anemia. Kidney damage might also be present. Treatment options include chemotherapy, targeted agents and immune modulators with or without bone marrow transplantation.

ILLUSTRATION BY PAM CURRY
ORIGINALLY PUBLISHED IN "FROM EVERY ANGLE," *CURE* SUMMER 2013

Ovarian Cancer

Following an ovarian cancer diagnosis, staging determines the best options for treatment, which may include surgery, chemotherapy or a combination of the two.

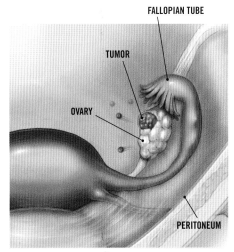

FALLOPIAN TUBE

TUMOR

OVARY

PERITONEUM

STAGE 1:

In addition to the presence of cancer cells in one or both ovaries (1A and 1B), cancer cells can be found on the surface of the ovary and in the surrounding fluid (1C).

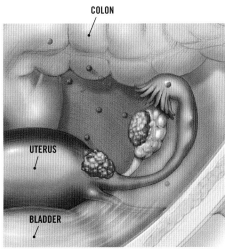

COLON

UTERUS

BLADDER

STAGE 2:

Cancer cells have spread to the surface of nearby tissues in the peritoneal cavity, including the fallopian tubes and/or uterus as well as the surrounding fluid.

TREATMENT OPTIONS:

SURGERY

CHEMOTHERAPY FOR HIGH-RISK DISEASE (STAGES 1C, 2)

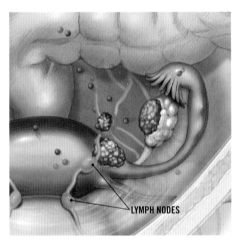

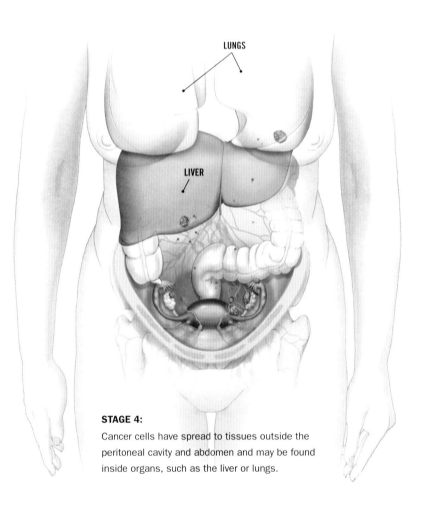

STAGE 3:

Cancer cells have spread to the nearby peritoneum and/or lymph nodes and may be present on the surface of tissues outside the peritoneal cavity, such as the liver.

STAGE 4:

Cancer cells have spread to tissues outside the peritoneal cavity and abdomen and may be found inside organs, such as the liver or lungs.

SURGERY (TO REDUCE TUMOR BULK) FOLLOWED BY CHEMOTHERAPY*

CHEMOTHERAPY FOLLOWED BY DEBULKING SURGERY, THEN CHEMOTHERAPY (STAGE 4)*

*Surgery may not be an option in some cases.

ILLUSTRATION BY ERIN MOORE
ORIGINALLY PUBLISHED IN "BREAKING OUT OF THE SILENCE," *CURE* SPRING 2011

Pleural Mesothelioma

[Unlike lung cancer, pleural mesothelioma begins in the lining of the lung. Treatment options depend on how far the disease has advanced, along with the tumor type.]

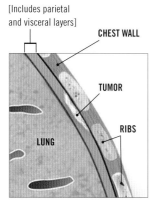

STAGE 1A: Tumor is confined to the parietal pleura, the external layer of the pleura.

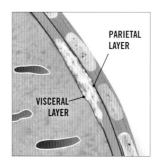

STAGE 1B: Tumor occupies the parietal pleura and the visceral pleura, the internal layer of the pleura that covers the lung.

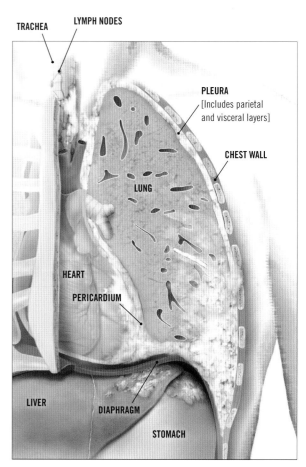

STAGE 4: Tumor invades multiple areas, penetrates the pericardium or diaphragm, extends into lymph nodes outside the chest and/or spreads to at least one other organ, such as the heart, esophagus, liver or opposite lung.

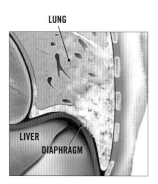

STAGE 2: Tumor expands into the lung or diaphragm.

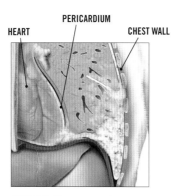

STAGE 3: Tumor extends into the chest wall, the tissue surrounding the heart (pericardium) and/or the lymph nodes in the chest.

CANCER STAGING

2

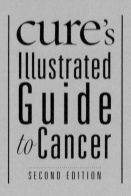

Chapter 3

Causes & Risks

CANCER CELLS emerge because of damage to DNA, the genetic blueprint that instructs cell growth. Usually the body is able to repair altered DNA, but in cancer cells, the damaged DNA cannot be repaired. In some cases, people inherit altered DNA, which may later cause cancer. More commonly, a person's DNA is changed by exposure to environmental factors or by random cellular events. For example, although most cases of lung cancer can be attributed to smoking, other risk factors may include having a lung disease such as chronic obstructive pulmonary disease, genetic susceptibility to lung cancer or exposure to secondhand smoke, radon gas, asbestos or other chemicals.

Lung Cancer in Never-Smokers

Lung cancer in never-smokers can be caused by environmental triggers, such as cooking fumes, secondhand smoke, asbestos, radon gas and various cancer-causing chemicals.

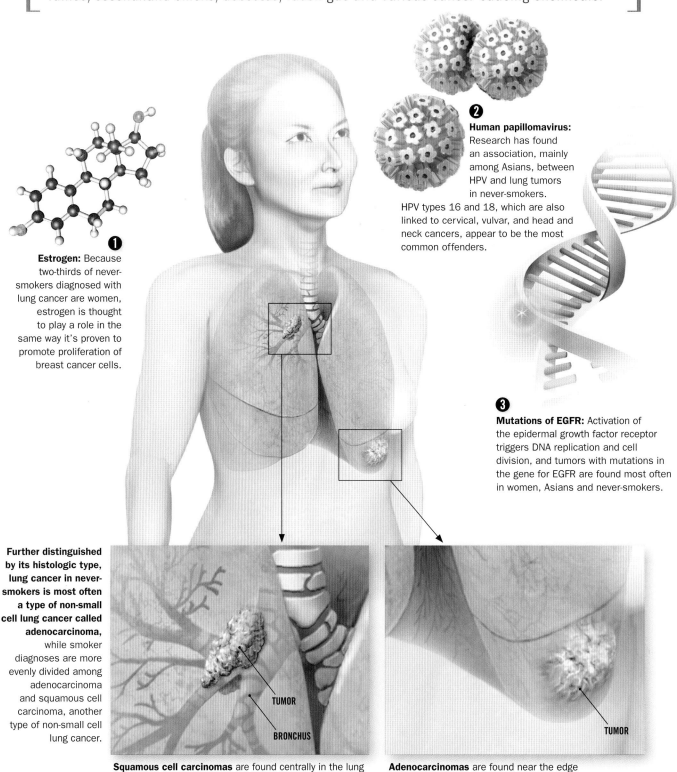

❶ **Estrogen:** Because two-thirds of never-smokers diagnosed with lung cancer are women, estrogen is thought to play a role in the same way it's proven to promote proliferation of breast cancer cells.

❷ **Human papillomavirus:** Research has found an association, mainly among Asians, between HPV and lung tumors in never-smokers. HPV types 16 and 18, which are also linked to cervical, vulvar, and head and neck cancers, appear to be the most common offenders.

❸ **Mutations of EGFR:** Activation of the epidermal growth factor receptor triggers DNA replication and cell division, and tumors with mutations in the gene for EGFR are found most often in women, Asians and never-smokers.

Further distinguished by its histologic type, lung cancer in never-smokers is most often a type of non-small cell lung cancer called adenocarcinoma, while smoker diagnoses are more evenly divided among adenocarcinoma and squamous cell carcinoma, another type of non-small cell lung cancer.

TUMOR

BRONCHUS

TUMOR

Squamous cell carcinomas are found centrally in the lung near the bronchi.

Adenocarcinomas are found near the edge of the lung.

CAUSES & RISKS

3

Evolution of Liver Cancer

Liver cancer, also known as hepatocellular carcinoma, can be caused by hepatitis B and C or chronic alcohol use.

 ❶

The trio of chronic alcohol consumption and hepatitis B and C, as well as other risk factors, can cause scarring of the liver, known as cirrhosis.

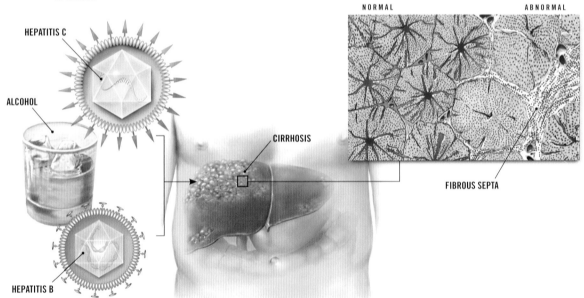

HEPATITIS C

ALCOHOL

CIRRHOSIS

HEPATITIS B

NORMAL   ABNORMAL

FIBROUS SEPTA

❷ The volume of fluid outside of cells, known as extracellular fluid, is maintained within narrow limits in healthy people. For people with cirrhosis, the extracellular fluid volume progressively builds up, **leading to inflammation and a buildup of the fibrous septa between the lobules.**

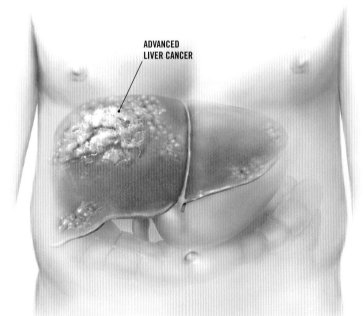

ADVANCED LIVER CANCER

❸

A cirrhotic liver has the ability to regenerate and repair damaged tissue, **but excessive cycles of liver cell death and renewal can cause permanent damage and lead to liver cancer**—a majority of which are diagnosed at an advanced stage.

ILLUSTRATION BY PAM CURRY
ORIGINALLY PUBLISHED IN "LIVER CANCER: MORE CASES, MORE CAUSES," *CURE* SPRING 2007

Inflammation

Chronic inflammation can trigger the immune system to battle against a persistent viral infection or bacterium, such as *H. pylori*, and can contribute to the development of cancer.

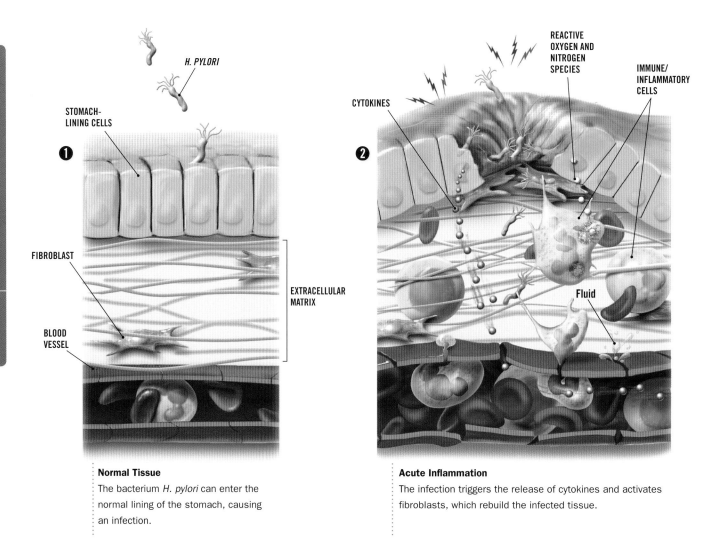

H. PYLORI

STOMACH-LINING CELLS

❶

FIBROBLAST

EXTRACELLULAR MATRIX

BLOOD VESSEL

REACTIVE OXYGEN AND NITROGEN SPECIES

IMMUNE/ INFLAMMATORY CELLS

CYTOKINES

❷

Fluid

Normal Tissue
The bacterium *H. pylori* can enter the normal lining of the stomach, causing an infection.

Acute Inflammation
The infection triggers the release of cytokines and activates fibroblasts, which rebuild the infected tissue.

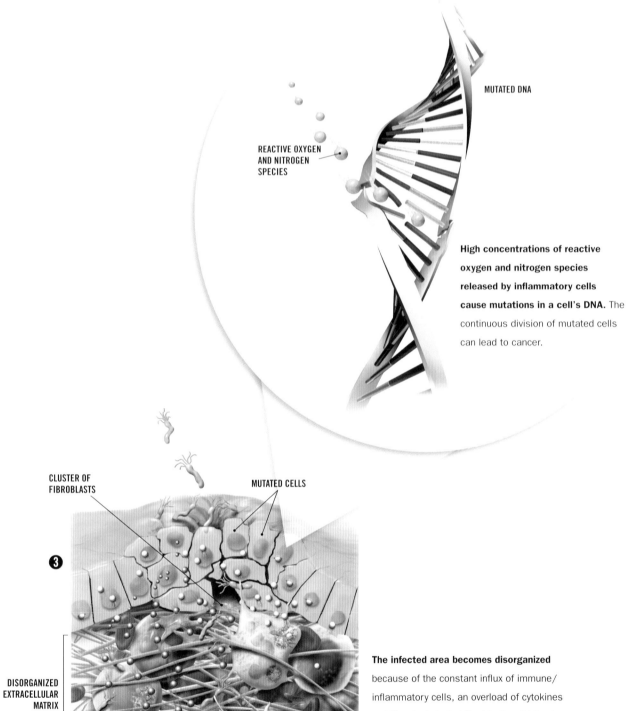

MUTATED DNA

REACTIVE OXYGEN AND NITROGEN SPECIES

High concentrations of reactive oxygen and nitrogen species released by inflammatory cells cause mutations in a cell's DNA. The continuous division of mutated cells can lead to cancer.

CLUSTER OF FIBROBLASTS

MUTATED CELLS

❸

DISORGANIZED EXTRACELLULAR MATRIX

The infected area becomes disorganized because of the constant influx of immune/ inflammatory cells, an overload of cytokines and the clustering of fibroblasts, which release extracellular matrix proteins that help cells survive and multiply.

Chronic Inflammation
Inflammation goes from acute to chronic if it doesn't resolve or becomes uncontrollable because of repeated tissue damage from the *H. pylori* infection or because of other disorders in the inflammatory process.

ILLUSTRATION BY PAM CURRY
ORIGINALLY PUBLISHED IN "THE INTERNAL FLAME," *CURE* FALL 2009

The Dangerous Path of Fat

[Although caused in some degree by inactivity, fat cells are not inactive. Here's how they harm the body.]

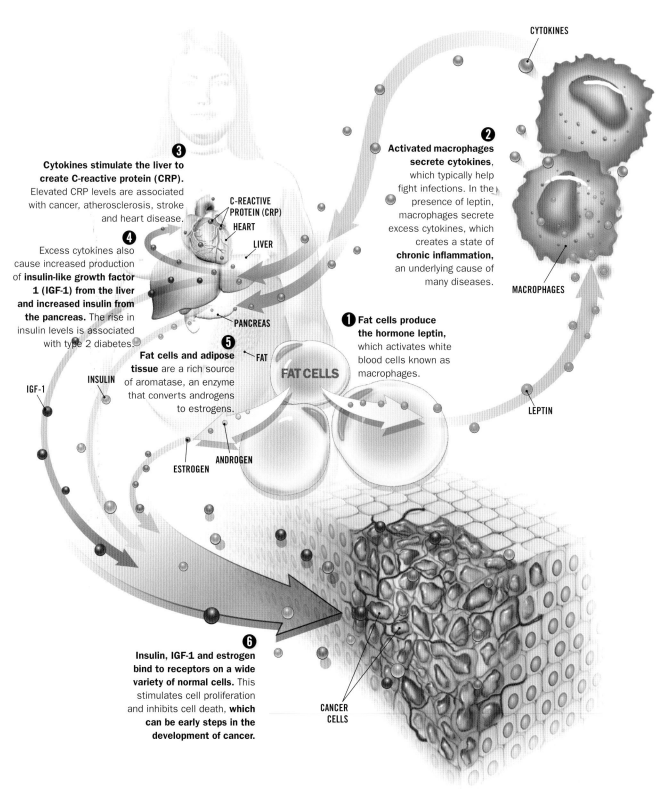

CYTOKINES

❸ **Cytokines stimulate the liver to create C-reactive protein (CRP).** Elevated CRP levels are associated with cancer, atherosclerosis, stroke and heart disease.

C-REACTIVE PROTEIN (CRP)

HEART

LIVER

❹ Excess cytokines also cause increased production of **insulin-like growth factor 1 (IGF-1) from the liver and increased insulin from the pancreas.** The rise in insulin levels is associated with type 2 diabetes.

PANCREAS

❷ **Activated macrophages secrete cytokines**, which typically help fight infections. In the presence of leptin, macrophages secrete excess cytokines, which creates a state of **chronic inflammation,** an underlying cause of many diseases.

MACROPHAGES

❶ **Fat cells produce the hormone leptin,** which activates white blood cells known as macrophages.

❺ **Fat cells and adipose tissue** are a rich source of aromatase, an enzyme that converts androgens to estrogens.

FAT

FAT CELLS

IGF-1

INSULIN

ESTROGEN

ANDROGEN

LEPTIN

❻ **Insulin, IGF-1 and estrogen bind to receptors on a wide variety of normal cells.** This stimulates cell proliferation and inhibits cell death, **which can be early steps in the development of cancer.**

CANCER CELLS

CAUSES & RISKS

3

ILLUSTRATION BY ERIN MOORE
ORIGINALLY PUBLISHED IN "ENERGY BALANCE," *CURE* FALL 2010

Estrogen's Effects

The effects of natural estrogen are seen throughout the body. Hormone replacement therapy may be used to sustain these effects but may also increase the risk of breast cancer growth.

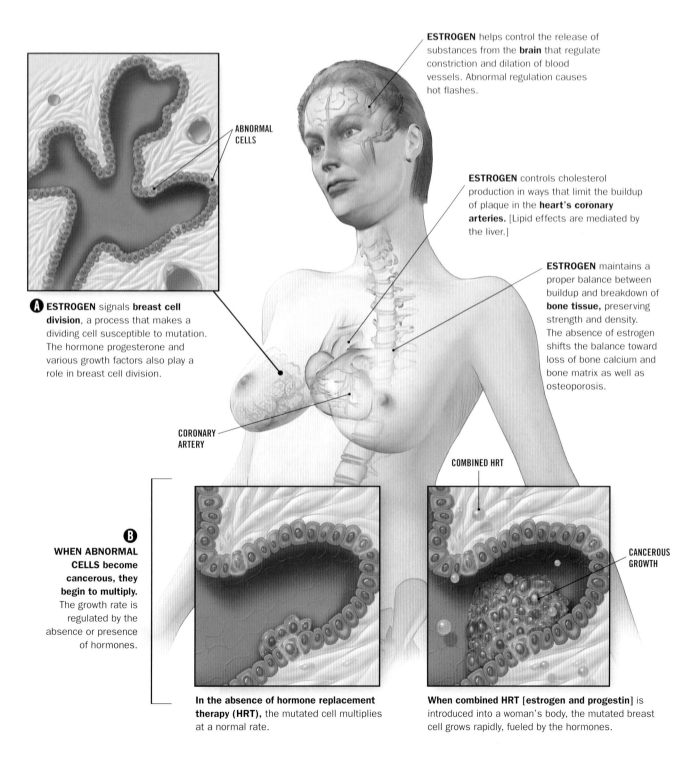

ESTROGEN helps control the release of substances from the **brain** that regulate constriction and dilation of blood vessels. Abnormal regulation causes hot flashes.

ESTROGEN controls cholesterol production in ways that limit the buildup of plaque in the **heart's coronary arteries.** [Lipid effects are mediated by the liver.]

ESTROGEN maintains a proper balance between buildup and breakdown of **bone tissue,** preserving strength and density. The absence of estrogen shifts the balance toward loss of bone calcium and bone matrix as well as osteoporosis.

ABNORMAL CELLS

A ESTROGEN signals **breast cell division**, a process that makes a dividing cell susceptible to mutation. The hormone progesterone and various growth factors also play a role in breast cell division.

CORONARY ARTERY

B WHEN ABNORMAL CELLS become cancerous, they begin to multiply. The growth rate is regulated by the absence or presence of hormones.

COMBINED HRT

CANCEROUS GROWTH

In the absence of hormone replacement therapy (HRT), the mutated cell multiplies at a normal rate.

When combined HRT [estrogen and progestin] is introduced into a woman's body, the mutated breast cell grows rapidly, fueled by the hormones.

ILLUSTRATION BY ERIN MOORE
ORIGINALLY PUBLISHED IN "THE HRT CONNECTION," *CURE* FALL 2007

Pleural Mesothelioma Cause and Effect

[
Pleural mesothelioma, a cancer that invades the lining of the lungs, is often caused by exposure to asbestos.
]

CAUSES

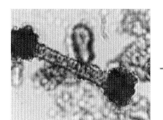

While asbestos is estimated to cause about 80 percent of mesothelioma cases, other causes are being studied.

DIAGNOSTIC

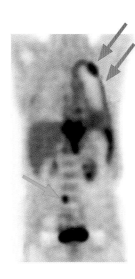

Positron emission tomography (PET) scan of a patient with stage 4 mesothelioma showing disease in the superior part of the lung (orange arrows) and a metastatic lesion in the abdomen (green arrow).

CAUSES & RISKS 3

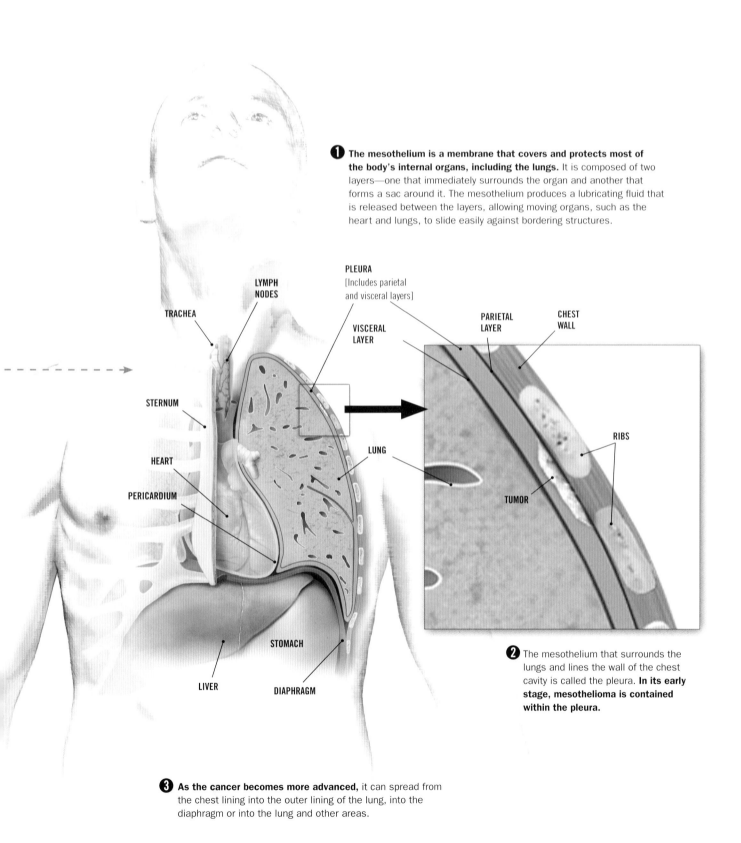

1 **The mesothelium is a membrane that covers and protects most of the body's internal organs, including the lungs.** It is composed of two layers—one that immediately surrounds the organ and another that forms a sac around it. The mesothelium produces a lubricating fluid that is released between the layers, allowing moving organs, such as the heart and lungs, to slide easily against bordering structures.

PLEURA
[Includes parietal and visceral layers]

LYMPH NODES

TRACHEA

VISCERAL LAYER

PARIETAL LAYER

CHEST WALL

STERNUM

RIBS

LUNG

HEART

TUMOR

PERICARDIUM

STOMACH

LIVER

DIAPHRAGM

2 The mesothelium that surrounds the lungs and lines the wall of the chest cavity is called the pleura. **In its early stage, mesothelioma is contained within the pleura.**

3 **As the cancer becomes more advanced,** it can spread from the chest lining into the outer lining of the lung, into the diaphragm or into the lung and other areas.

ILLUSTRATION BY PAM CURRY
ORIGINALLY PUBLISHED IN *UNDERSTANDING MESOTHELIOMA*, 2009

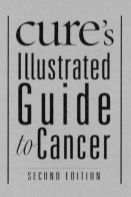

Chapter 4

Symptoms & Diagnosis

SYMPTOMS of cancer can range from being palpable, such as a lump, to vague, such as fatigue or pain. Some symptoms are specific to certain cancers. For example, blood in the urine or pain during urination may be signs of bladder cancer, but they could also be symptoms of other diseases, such as a urinary tract infection. Diagnostic tests help physicians confirm cancer and determine treatment. X-rays, CT scans and PET scans may be used to detect and stage cancer. A pathologist may examine blood samples or tissue from biopsies to diagnose cancer. There are other diagnostic tests available, and many new tests are being developed to help physicians identify, analyze and treat cancer.

Ovarian Cancer Symptoms

[As a tumor in the ovary spreads, it can cause a variety of symptoms that are specifically related to the tumor.]

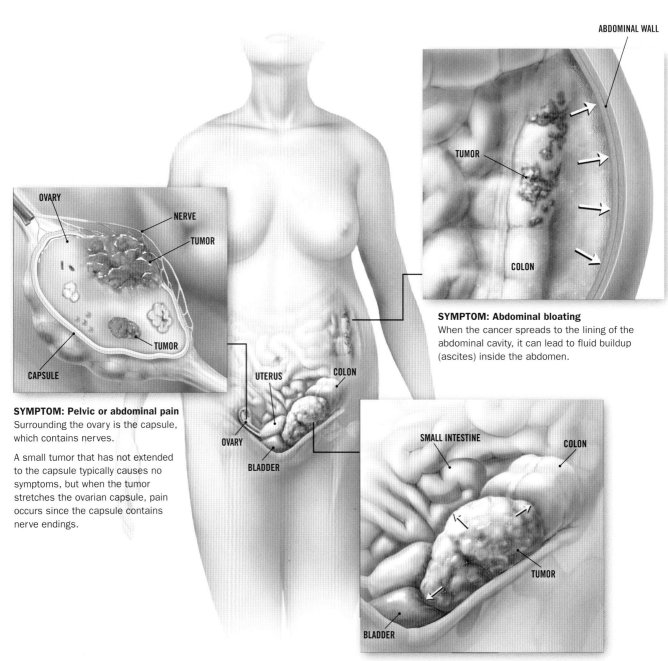

ABDOMINAL WALL

TUMOR

COLON

SYMPTOM: Abdominal bloating
When the cancer spreads to the lining of the abdominal cavity, it can lead to fluid buildup (ascites) inside the abdomen.

OVARY
NERVE
TUMOR
TUMOR
CAPSULE

UTERUS
COLON
OVARY
BLADDER

SYMPTOM: Pelvic or abdominal pain
Surrounding the ovary is the capsule, which contains nerves.

A small tumor that has not extended to the capsule typically causes no symptoms, but when the tumor stretches the ovarian capsule, pain occurs since the capsule contains nerve endings.

SMALL INTESTINE
COLON
TUMOR
BLADDER

SYMPTOMS: Urinary frequency or urgency and difficulty eating
An advanced tumor can block or thicken the intestinal tract, causing the patient to feel full too quickly after eating and to experience bloating and other abdominal symptoms.

Urinary frequency or urgency occurs when the tumor puts excessive pressure on the bladder.

ILLUSTRATION BY PAM CURRY
ORIGINALLY PUBLISHED IN "WARNING SIGNS," *CURE* WINTER 2007

Symptoms of Multiple Myeloma

A number of signs or symptoms related to multiple myeloma, such as fractures, bone pain, fatigue, swelling and weakness, may lead a patient to seek medical advice.

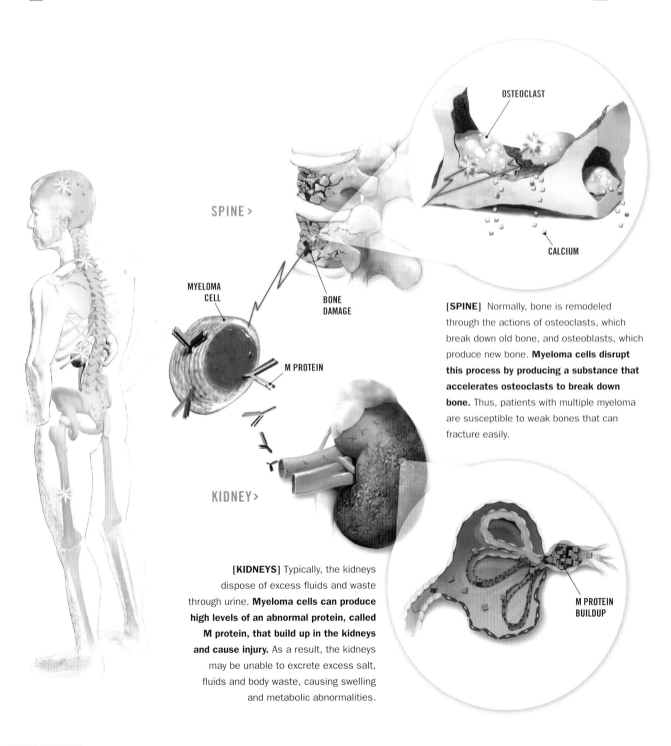

OSTEOCLAST

CALCIUM

SPINE >

MYELOMA CELL

BONE DAMAGE

M PROTEIN

KIDNEY >

M PROTEIN BUILDUP

[SPINE] Normally, bone is remodeled through the actions of osteoclasts, which break down old bone, and osteoblasts, which produce new bone. **Myeloma cells disrupt this process by producing a substance that accelerates osteoclasts to break down bone.** Thus, patients with multiple myeloma are susceptible to weak bones that can fracture easily.

[KIDNEYS] Typically, the kidneys dispose of excess fluids and waste through urine. **Myeloma cells can produce high levels of an abnormal protein, called M protein, that build up in the kidneys and cause injury.** As a result, the kidneys may be unable to excrete excess salt, fluids and body waste, causing swelling and metabolic abnormalities.

ILLUSTRATION BY PAM CURRY
ORIGINALLY PUBLISHED IN *CURE'S ILLUSTRATED GUIDE SECOND EDITION, 2013*

Symptoms of Peritoneal Mesothelioma

[As the tumors of peritoneal mesothelioma progress inside the lining of the abdomen, several symptoms may occur.]

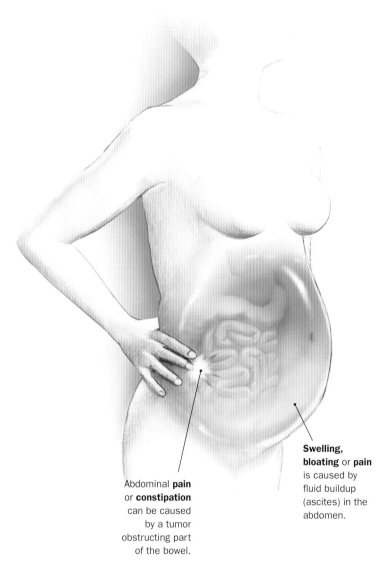

Abdominal **pain** or **constipation** can be caused by a tumor obstructing part of the bowel.

Swelling, bloating or **pain** is caused by fluid buildup (ascites) in the abdomen.

Disease Progression > While no established staging system exists at this time for peritoneal mesothelioma, here is how the disease may progress.

MESOTHELIUM
visceral layer -1
intramembrane space -2
parietal layer -3

MUSCLE
FAT
SKIN

COLON

1 2 3

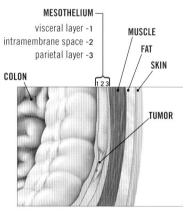

TUMOR

Tumor begins in the lining (mesothelium) covering the abdomen's internal organs. The tumor causes a thickening and an irritation of the lining.

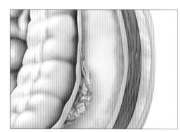

Tumor expands and results in fluid buildup in the abdomen.

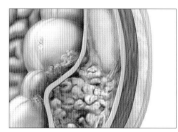

Tumor grows and penetrates the bowel, which can cause bowel obstruction and pain.

ILLUSTRATION BY PAM CURRY
ORIGINALLY PUBLISHED IN *UNDERSTANDING MESOTHELIOMA SECOND EDITION,* 2013

Cancers of Unknown Origin

[For patients diagnosed with metastatic cancer, the origin of the cancer may be difficult to detect. A variety of diagnostic tests can help doctors pinpoint where the cancer started.]

The first level of testing looks at the big picture

CT scan:
Provides a detailed cross-section image of parts of the body to locate tumors.

PET scan:
Detects tumors and determines how far the cancer has spread by measuring sugar absorption in the body's tissues.

Histology:
Based on how the cells look under the microscope, cancers are assigned to a subset with a specific treatment plan.

Chest X-ray:
Helps determine if cancer is present in the lung.

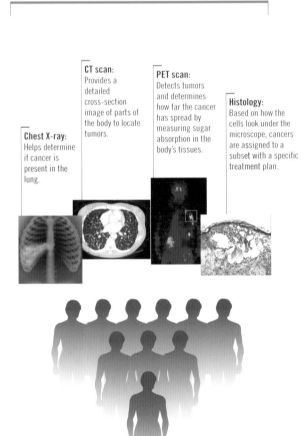

The second level takes an inside look at the cancer cells

Fluorescent in situ hybridization:
Uses fluorescent molecules to detect the number of cancer-related genes and their chromosomal positions in tumor cells.

Immuno-histochemistry:
A staining test that can identify cancer cells by the characteristic proteins on the cell surface and within the nucleus or cytoplasm.

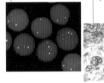

The third level involves tests that determine the genetic makeup of the cancer

Gene expression profiling:
Determines patterns of gene activity in the metastatic cancer and makes the best match based on typical patterns known for primary cancer of specific sites.

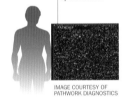

IMAGE COURTESY OF PATHWORK DIAGNOSTICS

Despite extensive testing, the origin of the cancer remains unknown in about 4 percent of patients.

ILLUSTRATION BY ERIN MOORE
ORIGINALLY PUBLISHED IN "NO I.D.," *CURE* SUMMER 2009

Diagnosing Sarcoma

Sarcoma develops in connective tissues, such as the bone, cartilage or muscle, and can be diagnosed with a variety of tests.

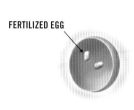

FERTILIZED EGG

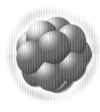

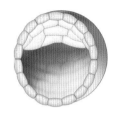

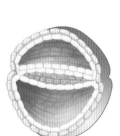

❶ SARCOMA develops from the cells that originate from the mesoderm, a germ layer that develops from the embryo along with the endoderm and ectoderm.

ECTODERM

MESODERM

ENDODERM

DIAGNOSIS OF SARCOMA involves a spectrum of tools. These techniques serve to confirm and subclassify the sarcoma type or to distinguish it from other cancers or benign scarring.

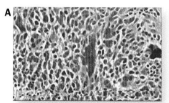

A

HISTOLOGY establishes a sarcoma diagnosis by examining the appearance of cancer cells under a microscope.

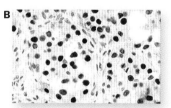

B

STANDARD IMMUNOHISTOCHEMISTRY, a widely used staining technique, can identify a specific protein within the nucleus, cytoplasm or on the surface of the cancer cell.

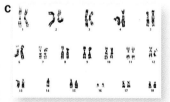

C

CHROMOSOMAL KARYOTYPING reveals chromosomal translocations and deletions indicative of certain types of sarcoma.

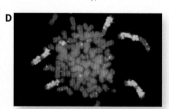

D

FLUORESCENT IN SITU HYBRIDIZATION [FISH], a more sensitive test than karyotype analysis, uses molecular probes to detect genetic abnormalities. Another more sensitive test, reverse transcriptase polymerase chain reaction [RT-PCR], detects small deletions and point mutations.

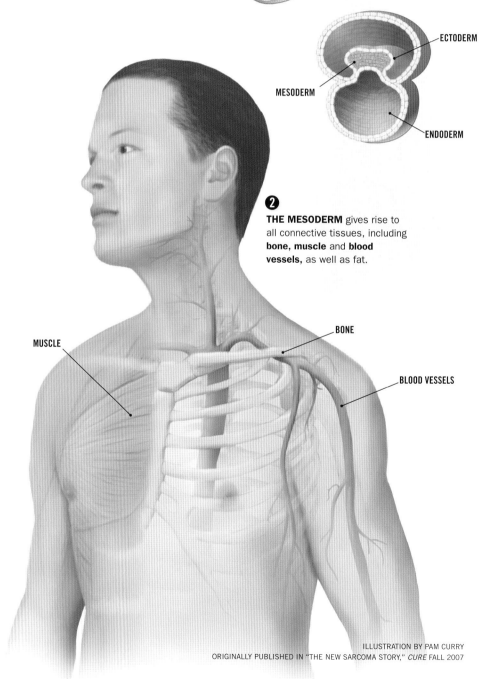

❷ THE MESODERM gives rise to all connective tissues, including **bone, muscle** and **blood vessels,** as well as fat.

MUSCLE

BONE

BLOOD VESSELS

Image A courtesy of Naseem Uddin, MD; Image B reprinted with permission from C.R. Antonescu, "The role of genetic testing in soft tissue sarcoma," *Histopathology,* 2006; Images C and D courtesy of Jonathan A. Fletcher, MD

ILLUSTRATION BY PAM CURRY
ORIGINALLY PUBLISHED IN "THE NEW SARCOMA STORY," *CURE* FALL 2007

Oncotype DX

Oncotype DX is a test that allows hormone-positive breast cancer patients to obtain a refined assessment that predicts their chance of recurrence and whether chemotherapy will reduce that risk.

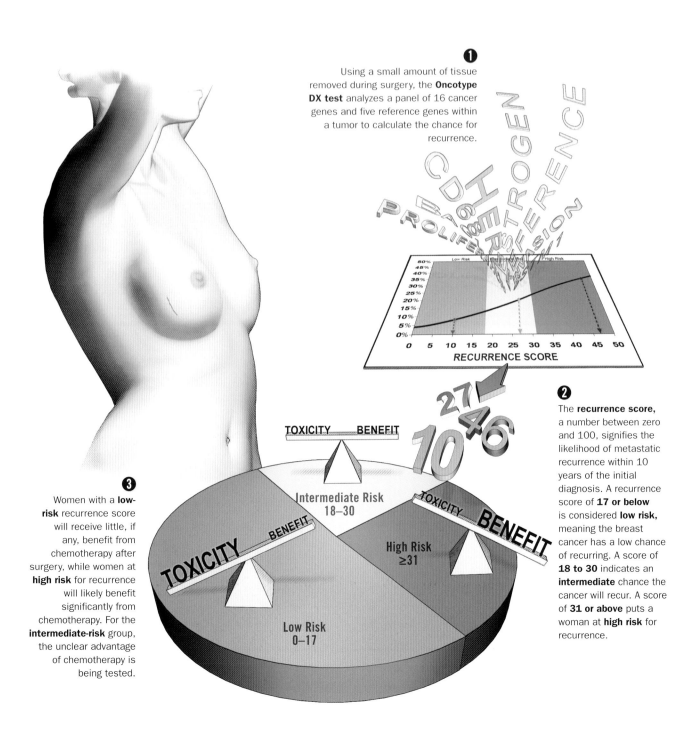

❶ Using a small amount of tissue removed during surgery, the **Oncotype DX test** analyzes a panel of 16 cancer genes and five reference genes within a tumor to calculate the chance for recurrence.

❷ The **recurrence score,** a number between zero and 100, signifies the likelihood of metastatic recurrence within 10 years of the initial diagnosis. A recurrence score of **17 or below** is considered **low risk,** meaning the breast cancer has a low chance of recurring. A score of **18 to 30** indicates an **intermediate** chance the cancer will recur. A score of **31 or above** puts a woman at **high risk** for recurrence.

❸ Women with a **low-risk** recurrence score will receive little, if any, benefit from chemotherapy after surgery, while women at **high risk** for recurrence will likely benefit significantly from chemotherapy. For the **intermediate-risk** group, the unclear advantage of chemotherapy is being tested.

ILLUSTRATION BY ERIN MOORE
ORIGINALLY PUBLISHED IN "FINDING YOUR COMPASS," *CURE* FALL 2008

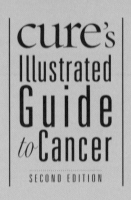

CURE's Illustrated Guide to Cancer
SECOND EDITION

Chapter 5

Treatments

TREATMENT for cancer may include surgery, radiation therapy, chemotherapy, hormonal therapy, stem cell transplantation, biological therapies or a combination of these treatments. In some cases, patients may have several treatment options. It is important that patients understand the possible benefits of each treatment, as well as the side effects and risks. Patients who have few options or want to try an experimental treatment may consider enrolling in a clinical trial. Clinical trials test new, experimental treatments to determine whether they are more effective than what is currently available, if they have fewer side effects or whether they are more convenient, such as medications taken by mouth or those with shorter treatment times. Some trials may offer standard therapy along with tests and new treatments. Search for clinical trials at curetoday.com/trialcheck.

Mohs Surgery

The Mohs technique is used to remove certain types of cancer, layer by layer, such as skin cancer.

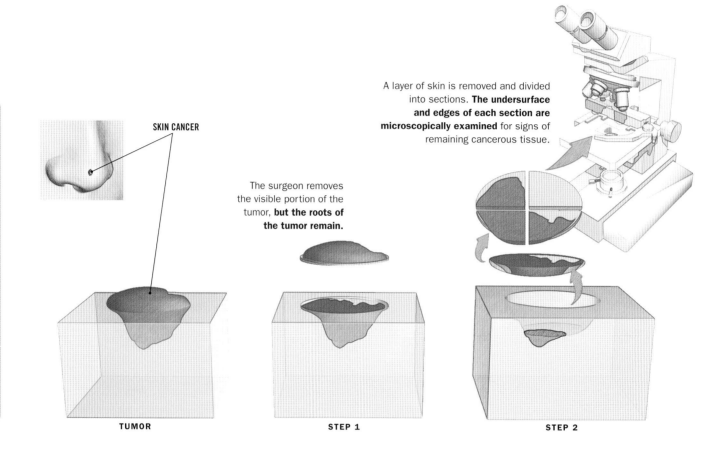

SKIN CANCER

A layer of skin is removed and divided into sections. **The undersurface and edges of each section are microscopically examined** for signs of remaining cancerous tissue.

The surgeon removes the visible portion of the tumor, **but the roots of the tumor remain.**

TUMOR

STEP 1

STEP 2

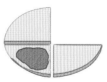

If cancerous tissue is seen under the microscope, **the surgeon removes another layer of skin** where the cancer cells remain.

The removal process is repeated **until microscopic evidence shows all cancerous tissue has been removed,** leaving healthy tissue undamaged.

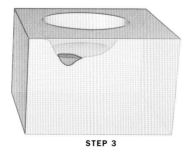

STEP 3

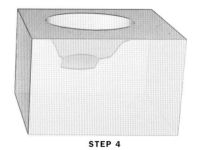

STEP 4

da Vinci Surgical System

[The da Vinci robot is a minimally invasive surgical technique that is used for a variety of procedures, including prostatectomy for prostate cancer.]

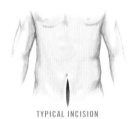

TYPICAL INCISION

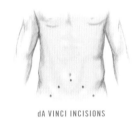

dA VINCI INCISIONS

IN TRADITIONAL prostate surgery, surgeons make an 8- to 10-inch incision on the lower abdomen versus **da Vinci's five 1- to 2-cm incisions,** which result in less blood loss.

❶

THE SURGEON leads the procedure from a console a few feet away from the patient. **The hand controls provide precise direction of the surgeon's movements,** filtering out hand tremors and translating large hand movements to micro-movements.

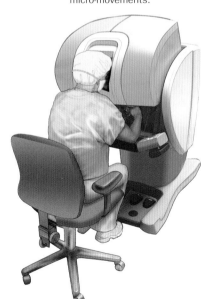

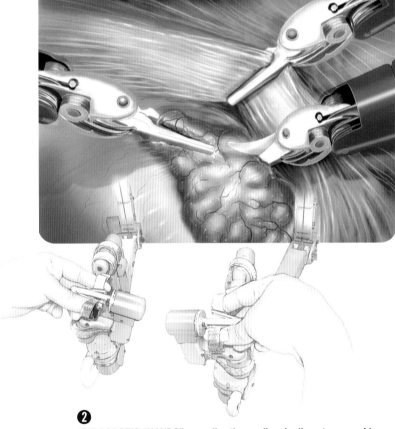

❷

THE ROBOT'S "HANDS"—smaller than a dime in diameter—provide a greater range of motion than the human hand to remove cancerous tissue from the prostate. After the tumor is separated from surrounding tissues, it's placed in a plastic pouch attached to a string, then pulled out through the middle incision near the navel.

ILLUSTRATION BY ERIN MOORE
ORIGINALLY PUBLISHED IN "SURGEONS & ROBOTS," *CURE* SUMMER 2007

Kidney Surgery

A partial nephrectomy is a surgical technique used to remove tumors from the kidney while preserving healthy tissue, as opposed to removing the entire kidney.

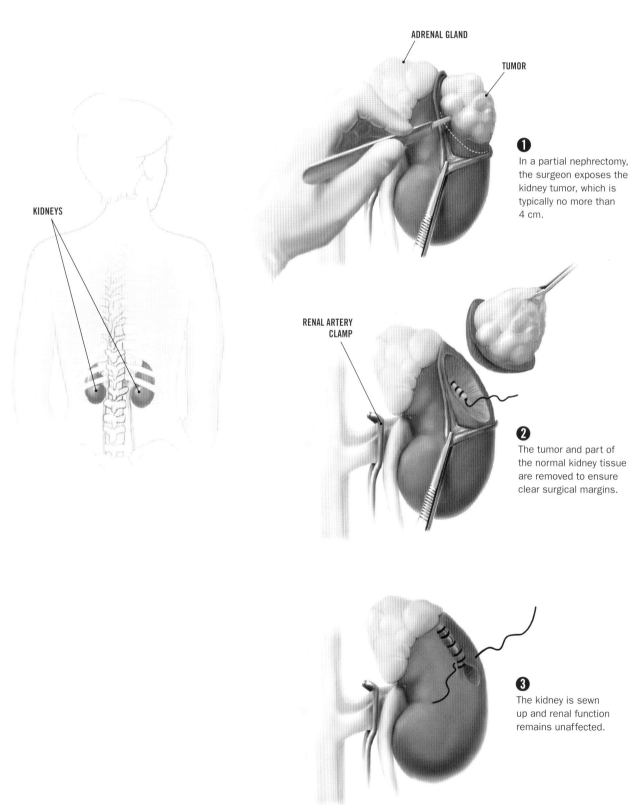

KIDNEYS

ADRENAL GLAND

TUMOR

❶ In a partial nephrectomy, the surgeon exposes the kidney tumor, which is typically no more than 4 cm.

RENAL ARTERY CLAMP

❷ The tumor and part of the normal kidney tissue are removed to ensure clear surgical margins.

❸ The kidney is sewn up and renal function remains unaffected.

ILLUSTRATION BY PAM CURRY
ORIGINALLY PUBLISHED IN "PICKING UP MOMENTUM," *CURE* SPRING 2006

TREATMENTS

5

Creating a New Bladder

Following a cystectomy (removal of the bladder), certain patients may receive a new bladder, also known as a neobladder, created from a section of the small intestine.

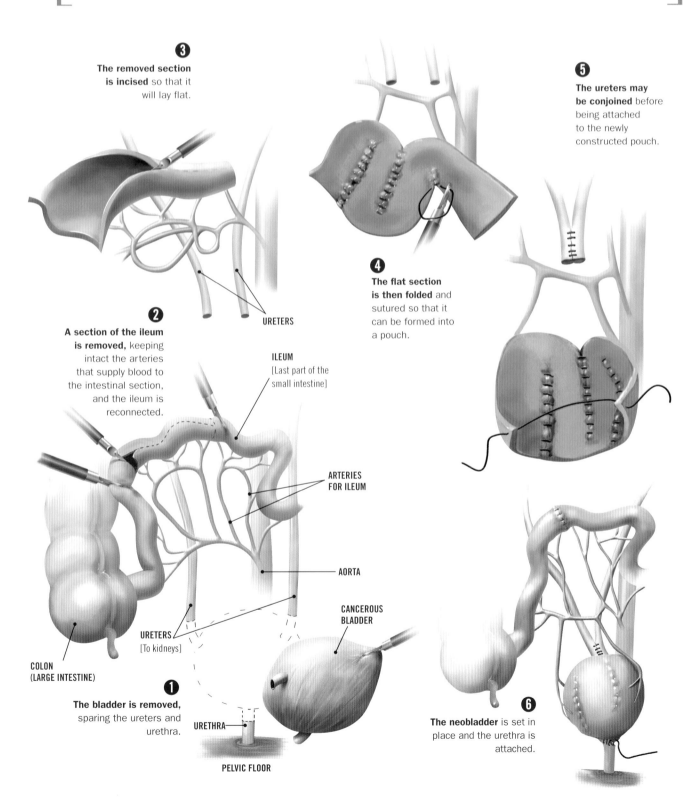

❸ The removed section is incised so that it will lay flat.

❺ The ureters may be conjoined before being attached to the newly constructed pouch.

❷ A section of the ileum is removed, keeping intact the arteries that supply blood to the intestinal section, and the ileum is reconnected.

URETERS

ILEUM
[Last part of the small intestine]

❹ The flat section is then folded and sutured so that it can be formed into a pouch.

ARTERIES FOR ILEUM

AORTA

CANCEROUS BLADDER

URETERS
[To kidneys]

COLON
(LARGE INTESTINE)

❶ The bladder is removed, sparing the ureters and urethra.

URETHRA

PELVIC FLOOR

❻ The neobladder is set in place and the urethra is attached.

ILLUSTRATION BY PAM CURRY
ORIGINALLY PUBLISHED IN "GOING THE DISTANCE," *CURE* SPRING 2012

Radiation Techniques

Compared to traditional radiation therapy, which can kill cancer cells but also damage healthy tissue, specialized techniques deliver radiation to the tumor more precisely.

TUMOR

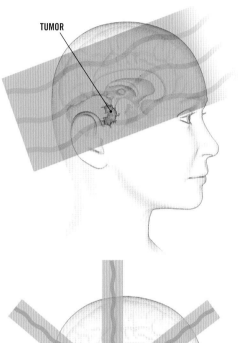

X-RAY BEAM

X-rays are high-energy photons (gamma rays) created by machines, and although the beam can be aimed at a tumor, the radiation dose is delivered to healthy tissue in front of and behind the tumor. The energy breaks DNA bonds, causing cell death.

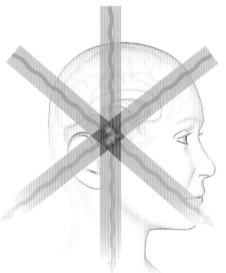

STEREOTACTIC RADIOSURGERY

Stereotactic radiosurgery uses highly focused gamma rays that originate at different angles and intersect at the tumor site. The tumor is hit with a high, concentrated dose of radiation, sparing the surrounding healthy tissue from the full dose.

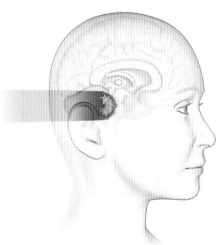

PROTON BEAM

The larger size of a proton particle, used in specific cases, ensures that the bulk of energy is deposited exactly at the tumor site, allowing more precise treatment and, in some cases, treatment of areas previously radiated with standard radiation.

ILLUSTRATION BY ERIN MOORE
ORIGINALLY PUBLISHED IN "A DIRECT HIT," *CURE SPECIAL ISSUE* 2008

Brachytherapy

Brachytherapy delivers radiation directly to the tumor site. Mammosite, depicted below, is specific for breast cancer and uses radioactive seeds.

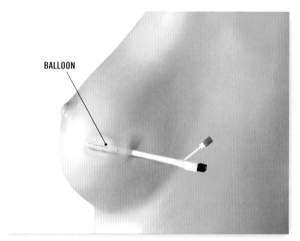

BALLOON

❶ A tube with a balloon attached to the end is inserted into the lumpectomy site.

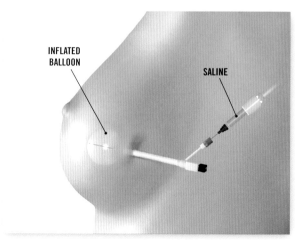

INFLATED BALLOON

SALINE

❷ The balloon is inflated and filled with saline.

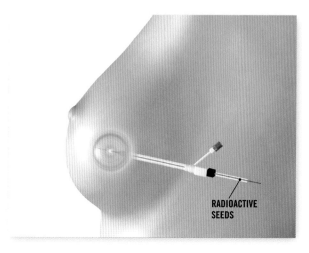

RADIOACTIVE SEEDS

❸ Radioactive "seeds" travel through the tube and into the balloon to deliver the radiation to kill remaining cancer cells. The balloon is deflated and removed after five days.

ILLUSTRATION BY ERIN MOORE
ORIGINALLY PUBLISHED IN "UNEXPECTED & UNIQUE," *CURE* FALL 2005

Stem Cell Transplantation

[Chemotherapy and radiation used to treat some cancers can damage stem cells. Stem cell transplantations introduce healthy cells back into the body.]

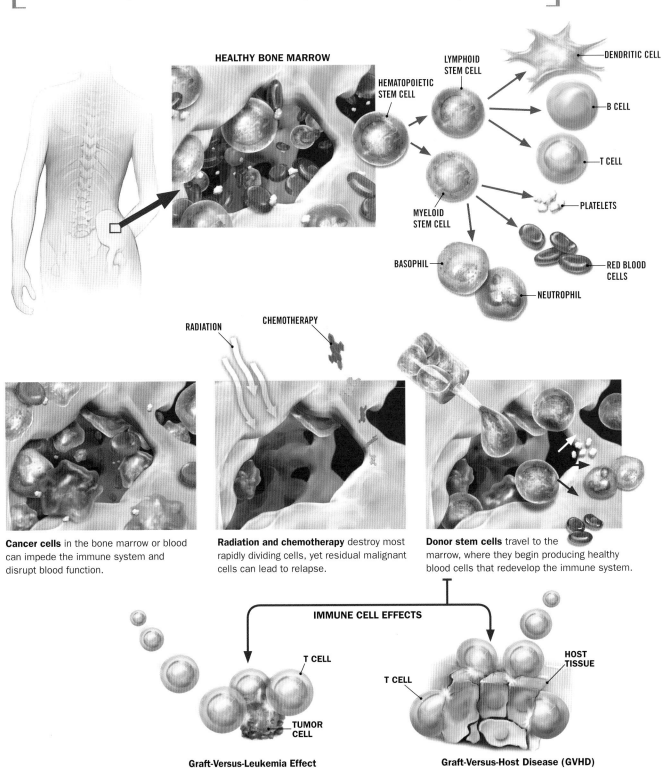

HEALTHY BONE MARROW

HEMATOPOIETIC STEM CELL

LYMPHOID STEM CELL

DENDRITIC CELL

B CELL

T CELL

PLATELETS

MYELOID STEM CELL

BASOPHIL

RED BLOOD CELLS

NEUTROPHIL

RADIATION

CHEMOTHERAPY

Cancer cells in the bone marrow or blood can impede the immune system and disrupt blood function.

Radiation and chemotherapy destroy most rapidly dividing cells, yet residual malignant cells can lead to relapse.

Donor stem cells travel to the marrow, where they begin producing healthy blood cells that redevelop the immune system.

IMMUNE CELL EFFECTS

T CELL

TUMOR CELL

HOST TISSUE

T CELL

Graft-Versus-Leukemia Effect
The donor immune cells (the graft) attack any remaining tumor cells in the blood (leukemia).

Graft-Versus-Host Disease (GVHD)
The donor immune cells (the graft) recognize the recipient's (the host's) tissues as "foreign" and attack those tissues.

ILLUSTRATION BY PAM CURRY
ORIGINALLY PUBLISHED IN "RISK VS. REWARD," *CURE* WINTER 2012

Targeted Therapies

Cancer cells develop certain characteristics that allow them to grow and survive.
These traits serve as the targets for a variety of cancer drugs.

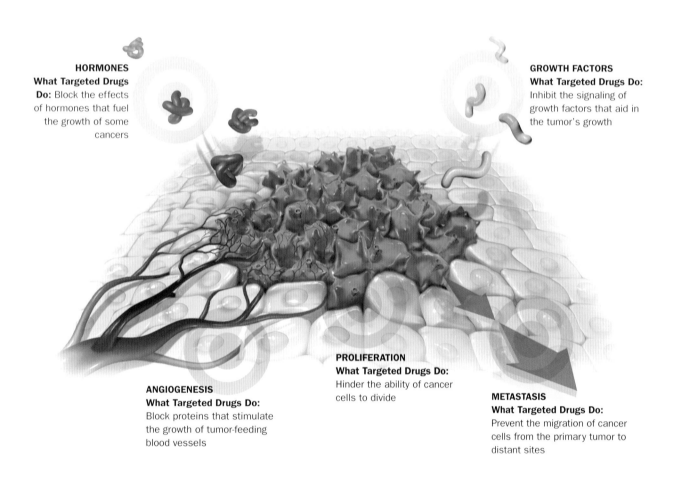

HORMONES
What Targeted Drugs Do: Block the effects of hormones that fuel the growth of some cancers

GROWTH FACTORS
What Targeted Drugs Do: Inhibit the signaling of growth factors that aid in the tumor's growth

ANGIOGENESIS
What Targeted Drugs Do: Block proteins that stimulate the growth of tumor-feeding blood vessels

PROLIFERATION
What Targeted Drugs Do: Hinder the ability of cancer cells to divide

METASTASIS
What Targeted Drugs Do: Prevent the migration of cancer cells from the primary tumor to distant sites

THE DIFFERENCE BETWEEN **CHEMOTHERAPY** AND **OTHER TARGETED DRUGS:**

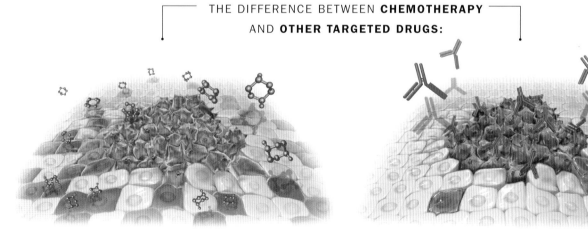

CHEMOTHERAPY targets and kills not only rapidly dividing cancer cells but also dividing healthy cells, such as hair follicles.

TARGETED AGENTS, such as monoclonal antibodies, specifically target and kill cancer cells while sparing most healthy cells.

ILLUSTRATION BY ERIN MOORE
ORIGINALLY PUBLISHED IN "TARGETED THERAPY: HOPE OR HYPE?" *CURE* SUMMER 2009

Tailoring Breast Cancer Treatments

Two breast cancer patients with very similar diagnoses may receive different local and systemic therapy. Here's an example of how treatment courses may differ based on different risk factors.

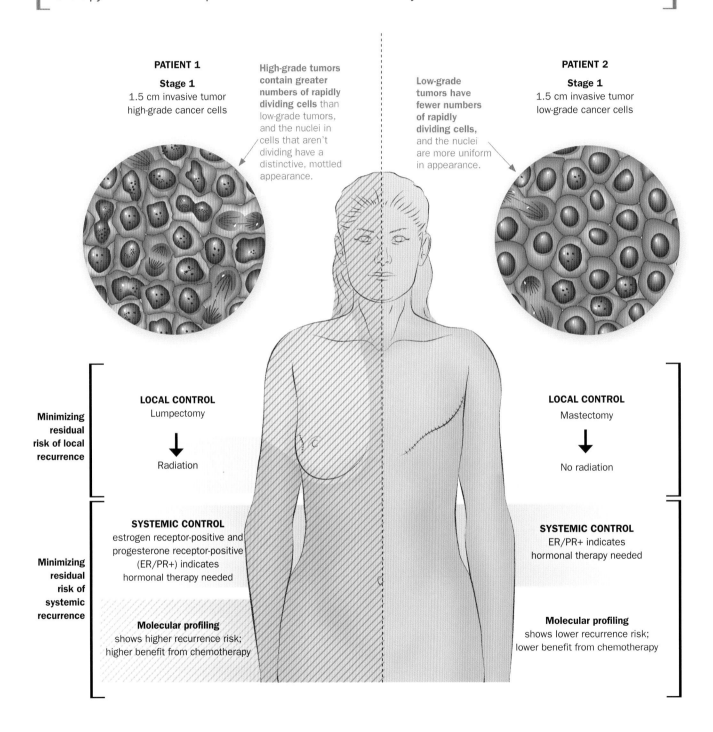

PATIENT 1

Stage 1

1.5 cm invasive tumor high-grade cancer cells

High-grade tumors contain greater numbers of rapidly dividing cells than low-grade tumors, and the nuclei in cells that aren't dividing have a distinctive, mottled appearance.

Low-grade tumors have fewer numbers of rapidly dividing cells, and the nuclei are more uniform in appearance.

PATIENT 2

Stage 1

1.5 cm invasive tumor low-grade cancer cells

Minimizing residual risk of local recurrence

LOCAL CONTROL
Lumpectomy
↓
Radiation

LOCAL CONTROL
Mastectomy
↓
No radiation

Minimizing residual risk of systemic recurrence

SYSTEMIC CONTROL
estrogen receptor-positive and progesterone receptor-positive (ER/PR+) indicates hormonal therapy needed

SYSTEMIC CONTROL
ER/PR+ indicates hormonal therapy needed

Molecular profiling
shows higher recurrence risk; higher benefit from chemotherapy

Molecular profiling
shows lower recurrence risk; lower benefit from chemotherapy

ILLUSTRATION BY ERIN MOORE
ORIGINALLY PUBLISHED IN "ONE DIAGNOSIS, DIFFERENT JOURNEYS," *CURE* FALL 2010

5 | TREATMENTS

Breast Cancer Treatments

Certain drugs target estrogen receptor-positive or HER2-positive breast cancers.
Research is examining whether better drugs or combinations can improve outcomes.

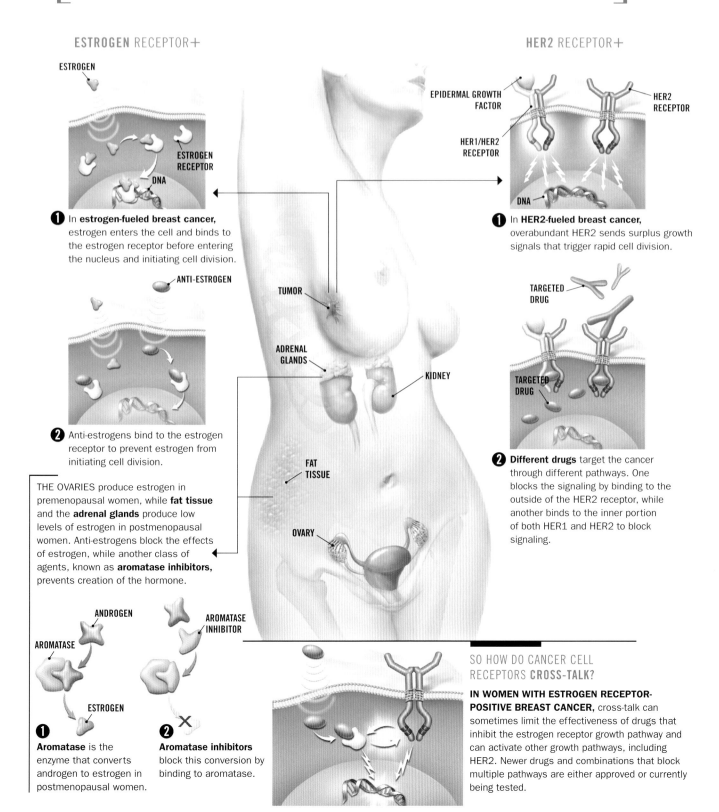

ESTROGEN RECEPTOR+

ESTROGEN

ESTROGEN RECEPTOR

DNA

1 In **estrogen-fueled breast cancer,** estrogen enters the cell and binds to the estrogen receptor before entering the nucleus and initiating cell division.

ANTI-ESTROGEN

2 Anti-estrogens bind to the estrogen receptor to prevent estrogen from initiating cell division.

THE OVARIES produce estrogen in premenopausal women, while **fat tissue** and the **adrenal glands** produce low levels of estrogen in postmenopausal women. Anti-estrogens block the effects of estrogen, while another class of agents, known as **aromatase inhibitors,** prevents creation of the hormone.

ANDROGEN

AROMATASE

AROMATASE INHIBITOR

ESTROGEN

1 Aromatase is the enzyme that converts androgen to estrogen in postmenopausal women.

2 Aromatase inhibitors block this conversion by binding to aromatase.

HER2 RECEPTOR+

EPIDERMAL GROWTH FACTOR

HER2 RECEPTOR

HER1/HER2 RECEPTOR

DNA

1 In **HER2-fueled breast cancer,** overabundant HER2 sends surplus growth signals that trigger rapid cell division.

TARGETED DRUG

TARGETED DRUG

2 Different drugs target the cancer through different pathways. One blocks the signaling by binding to the outside of the HER2 receptor, while another binds to the inner portion of both HER1 and HER2 to block signaling.

TUMOR

ADRENAL GLANDS

KIDNEY

FAT TISSUE

OVARY

SO HOW DO CANCER CELL RECEPTORS CROSS-TALK?

IN WOMEN WITH ESTROGEN RECEPTOR-POSITIVE BREAST CANCER, cross-talk can sometimes limit the effectiveness of drugs that inhibit the estrogen receptor growth pathway and can activate other growth pathways, including HER2. Newer drugs and combinations that block multiple pathways are either approved or currently being tested.

ILLUSTRATION BY PAM CURRY
ORIGINALLY PUBLISHED IN "A NEW ERA," *CURE SPECIAL ISSUE: ADVANCES IN BREAST CANCER* 2007

Anti-Estrogens

The hormone estrogen can drive the growth of some forms of breast cancer.
Anti-estrogens work to keep this at bay.

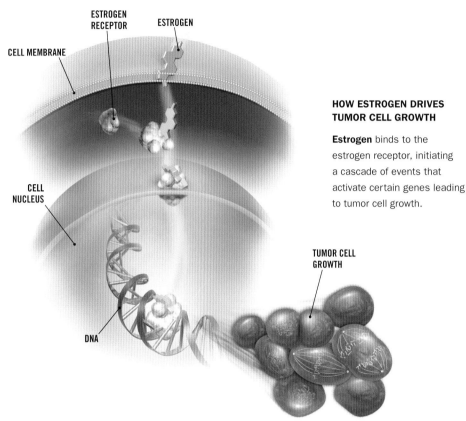

CELL MEMBRANE

ESTROGEN
RECEPTOR

ESTROGEN

CELL
NUCLEUS

DNA

TUMOR CELL
GROWTH

HOW ESTROGEN DRIVES TUMOR CELL GROWTH

Estrogen binds to the estrogen receptor, initiating a cascade of events that activate certain genes leading to tumor cell growth.

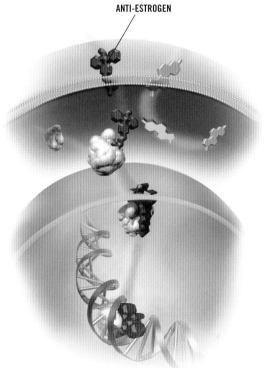

ANTI-ESTROGEN

HOW AN ANTI-ESTROGEN BLOCKS TUMOR GROWTH

An anti-estrogen blocks estrogen from binding to the estrogen receptor, disrupting the process that leads to tumor growth.

ILLUSTRATION BY PAM CURRY
ORIGINALLY PUBLISHED IN "THE ESTROGEN EFFECT," *CURE* FALL 2012

TREATMENTS

5

PARP Inhibitors

PARP inhibitors block an enzyme that repairs DNA damage and are effective against breast and ovarian cancers with BRCA1 and BRCA2 gene mutations.

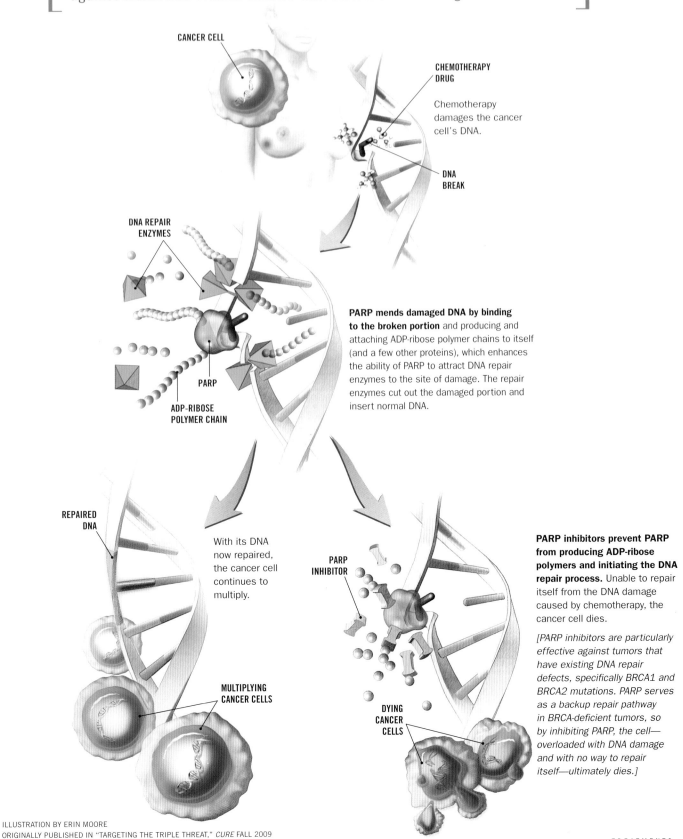

CANCER CELL

CHEMOTHERAPY DRUG

Chemotherapy damages the cancer cell's DNA.

DNA BREAK

DNA REPAIR ENZYMES

PARP

ADP-RIBOSE POLYMER CHAIN

PARP mends damaged DNA by binding to the broken portion and producing and attaching ADP-ribose polymer chains to itself (and a few other proteins), which enhances the ability of PARP to attract DNA repair enzymes to the site of damage. The repair enzymes cut out the damaged portion and insert normal DNA.

REPAIRED DNA

With its DNA now repaired, the cancer cell continues to multiply.

MULTIPLYING CANCER CELLS

PARP INHIBITOR

PARP inhibitors prevent PARP from producing ADP-ribose polymers and initiating the DNA repair process. Unable to repair itself from the DNA damage caused by chemotherapy, the cancer cell dies.

[PARP inhibitors are particularly effective against tumors that have existing DNA repair defects, specifically BRCA1 and BRCA2 mutations. PARP serves as a backup repair pathway in BRCA-deficient tumors, so by inhibiting PARP, the cell—overloaded with DNA damage and with no way to repair itself—ultimately dies.]

DYING CANCER CELLS

ILLUSTRATION BY ERIN MOORE
ORIGINALLY PUBLISHED IN "TARGETING THE TRIPLE THREAT," *CURE* FALL 2009

Targeting Notch

Some therapies take aim at notch signaling pathways in cancer stem cells. Characterized by asymmetrical division, these primitive and elusive cells can either remain dormant for long periods of time or mature into "regular" cancer cells.

❶ STEM CELL DIVISION ›
SELF-RENEWAL is a key property of stem cells, meaning **they can divide and make copies of themselves** without differentiation.

❷ NOTCH SIGNALING PATHWAY ›
FOR NOTCH to determine the cell's fate, **a notch ligand must bind to the extracellular portion of notch.** This signals the intracellular portion of notch to be clipped by an enzyme called gamma secretase.

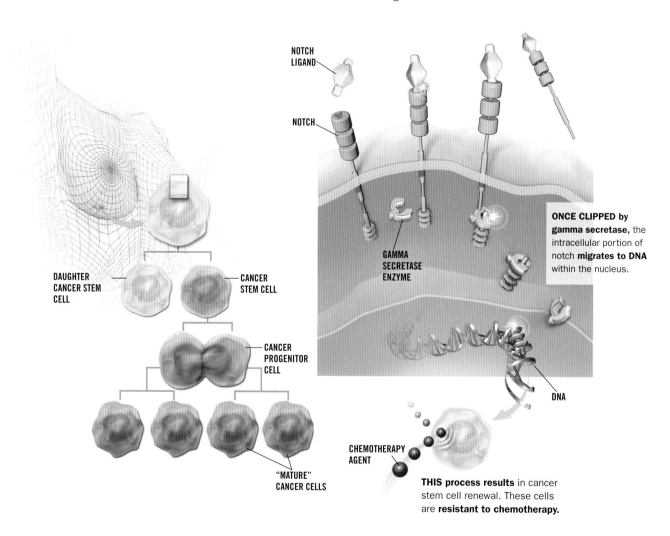

DAUGHTER CANCER STEM CELL

CANCER STEM CELL

CANCER PROGENITOR CELL

"MATURE" CANCER CELLS

NOTCH LIGAND

NOTCH

GAMMA SECRETASE ENZYME

ONCE CLIPPED by gamma secretase, the intracellular portion of notch **migrates to DNA** within the nucleus.

DNA

CHEMOTHERAPY AGENT

THIS process results in cancer stem cell renewal. These cells are **resistant to chemotherapy.**

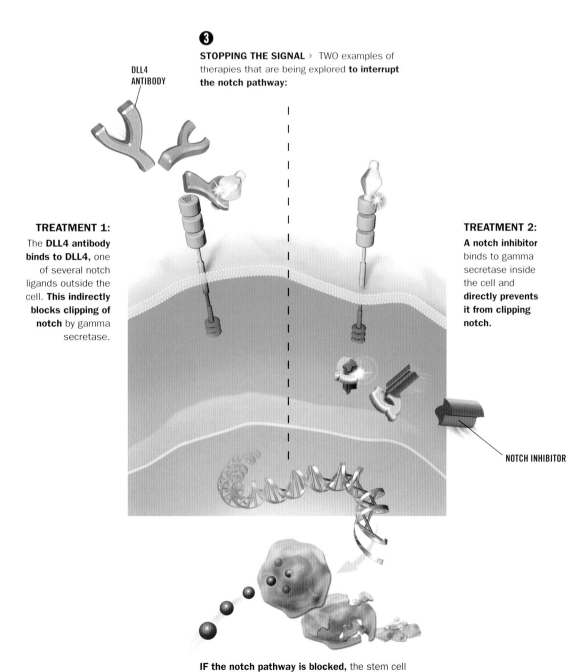

③

STOPPING THE SIGNAL › TWO examples of therapies that are being explored **to interrupt the notch pathway:**

DLL4 ANTIBODY

TREATMENT 1:
The **DLL4 antibody binds to DLL4,** one of several notch ligands outside the cell. **This indirectly blocks clipping of notch** by gamma secretase.

TREATMENT 2:
A notch inhibitor binds to gamma secretase inside the cell and **directly prevents it from clipping notch.**

NOTCH INHIBITOR

IF the notch pathway is blocked, the stem cell is directed to differentiate and the resulting cancer cells become **susceptible to chemotherapy.**

Brain Tumor Treatments

The tricky goal of gaining access to brain tumors has led to some unique approaches for treating cancer in the body's most complex organ.

❶ DIRECT EFFECT

The brain tumor has been surgically removed.

Treatment ›

Biopolymer wafers are placed inside the resection area to deliver chemotherapy to the surrounding brain tissue. The risk of common complications, such as seizures and cerebral edema, has made this treatment option less desirable.

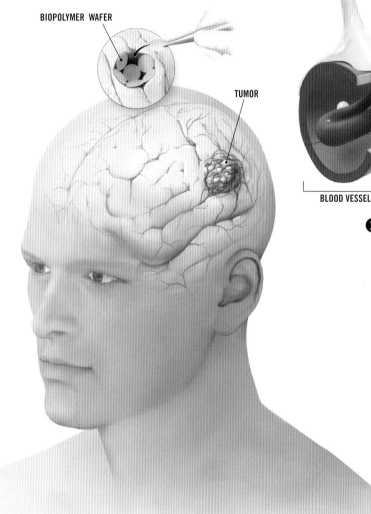

BIOPOLYMER WAFER

TUMOR

TUMOR

ASTROCYTE

ENDOTHELIAL CELLS

CHEMOTHERAPY

BLOOD VESSEL

❷ CROSSING THE BARRIER

The blood-brain barrier consists of tightly packed endothelial cells in brain capillaries and specialized brain cells called astrocytes.

Treatment ›

Because of their molecular structure, some chemotherapies are able to pass through cell membranes to reach the tumor. Many other drugs are either too large or have a natural structure-related electrical charge that does not allow them to penetrate the membrane.

TREATMENTS

5

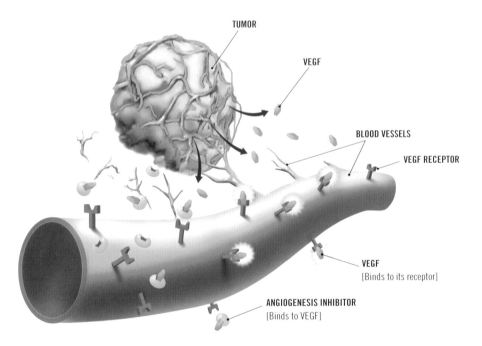

TUMOR

VEGF

BLOOD VESSELS

VEGF RECEPTOR

VEGF
[Binds to its receptor]

ANGIOGENESIS INHIBITOR
[Binds to VEGF]

❸ STARVING THE TUMOR

The formation of new blood vessels to supply the tumor with oxygen and nutrients is caused by a process called angiogenesis.

Treatment ›

Vascular endothelial growth factor [VEGF], a protein secreted by the tumor, binds to its receptor on endothelial cells that line blood vessel walls. Certain therapies, called angiogenesis inhibitors, can attach to VEGF and block this binding, thus stopping angiogenesis.

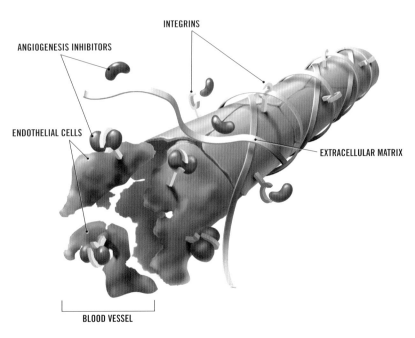

ANGIOGENESIS INHIBITORS

INTEGRINS

ENDOTHELIAL CELLS

EXTRACELLULAR MATRIX

BLOOD VESSEL

❹ CUTTING OFF THE BLOOD SUPPLY

Endothelial cells express integrins (protein receptors), which interact with the extracellular matrix and other endothelial cells to maintain the integrity of blood vessels.

Treatment ›

Some angiogenesis inhibitors are designed to bind to integrins, which in turn release their hold on the extracellular matrix, causing the blood vessels feeding the tumor to fall apart. Others bind the VEGF receptor and other angiogenic receptors or factors.

ILLUSTRATION BY PAM CURRY
ORIGINALLY PUBLISHED IN "A BETTER WAY TO THE BRAIN," *CURE* SUMMER 2008

Thyroid Cancer Treatment

> The thyroid gland naturally absorbs nearly all the iodine in the blood. Radioactive iodine therapy takes advantage of this to kill cancerous cells without affecting the rest of the body.

The Feedback Loop:

The hypothalamus produces thyrotropin-releasing hormone (TRH), which stimulates the pituitary gland to make thyroid-stimulating hormone (TSH).

①

HYPOTHALAMUS

PITUITARY GLAND

TRH

④

THYROID HORMONES

TSH

The hypothalamus senses the level of thyroid hormones in the body and mediates a feedback loop.

Low levels of thyroid hormones stimulate the production of TRH and subsequently higher levels of TSH and thyroid hormones.

High levels of thyroid hormones inhibit the production of TRH, which lowers TSH, thereby regulating thyroid function.

THYROID GLAND

THYROID HORMONES

②

TSH is transported via the blood to the thyroid gland.

③

TSH causes the thyroid gland to produce thyroid hormones needed to regulate the body's metabolism.

How Radioactive Iodine Therapy Works:

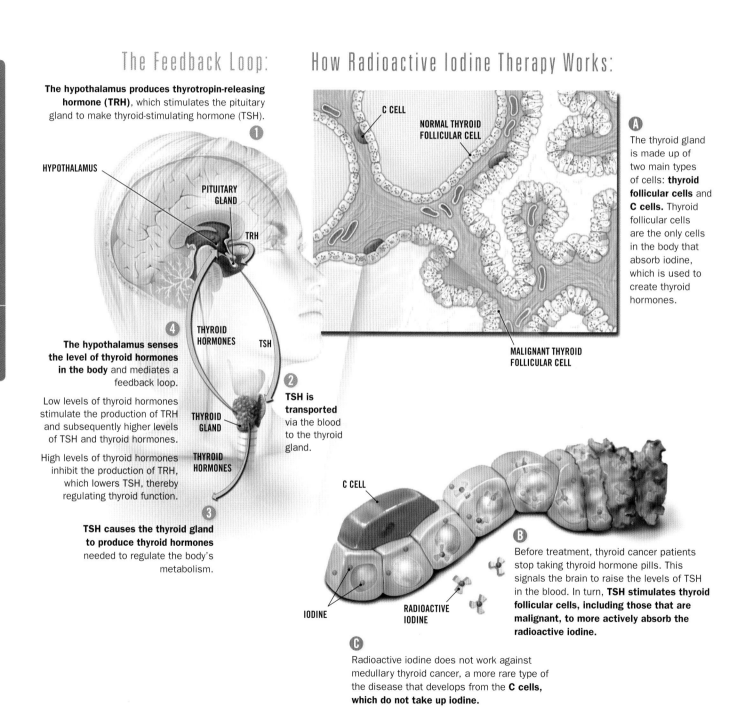

C CELL

NORMAL THYROID FOLLICULAR CELL

MALIGNANT THYROID FOLLICULAR CELL

Ⓐ The thyroid gland is made up of two main types of cells: **thyroid follicular cells** and **C cells.** Thyroid follicular cells are the only cells in the body that absorb iodine, which is used to create thyroid hormones.

C CELL

IODINE

RADIOACTIVE IODINE

Ⓑ Before treatment, thyroid cancer patients stop taking thyroid hormone pills. This signals the brain to raise the levels of TSH in the blood. In turn, **TSH stimulates thyroid follicular cells, including those that are malignant, to more actively absorb the radioactive iodine.**

Ⓒ Radioactive iodine does not work against medullary thyroid cancer, a more rare type of the disease that develops from the **C cells, which do not take up iodine.**

ILLUSTRATION BY PAM CURRY
ORIGINALLY PUBLISHED IN "THE GOOD CANCER?" *CURE* SPRING 2009

Kidney Cancer Treatments

The current arsenal of kidney cancer drugs includes immunotherapy, mTOR inhibitors and angiogenesis inhibitors.

1 Immunotherapy

Triggers the body's natural immune response to fight cancer

(A) Stimulatory cytokines activate and boost the production of cytotoxic T cells.

CANCER CELLS

STIMULATORY CYTOKINE

T CELL

(B) Cytotoxic T cells seek out and destroy the cancer.

CYTOTOXIC T CELL

2 mTOR Inhibitors

Turn off the signals that tell the cancer cell and blood vessel cells to grow

GROWTH FACTORS BIND TO RECEPTORS

mTOR INHIBITOR

CANCER CELL

mTOR

HIF-1

Proliferation

Angiogenesis

SIGNALING PATHWAYS

(A) The protein mTOR plays a key role in signaling the cancer cell to grow and survive.

(B) mTOR inhibitors block the mTOR pathway and prevent cancer growth.

3 Angiogenesis Inhibitors

Starve the tumor by cutting off its blood supply

(A) Vascular endothelial growth factor [VEGF] is a protein produced by the tumor.

VEGF

CANCER CELLS

VEGF BINDS TO ITS RECEPTOR

ANGIOGENESIS INHIBITOR

(B) The binding of VEGF to its receptor stimulates the formation of new blood vessels that supply the tumor with nutrients and oxygen.

ANGIOGENESIS INHIBITOR BINDS TO VEGF

(C) Some angiogenesis inhibitors work by blocking the growth signal from inside the cell by binding to the tyrosine kinase portion of the VEGF receptor.

(D) Other angiogenesis inhibitors work by attaching to VEGF and preventing the protein from binding to its receptor.

GROWTH SIGNAL

ANGIOGENESIS INHIBITOR

ILLUSTRATION BY PAM CURRY
ORIGINALLY PUBLISHED IN "REINING IN RENAL CANCER," *CURE* SUMMER 2009

Non-Hodgkin Lymphoma Treatments

Cell division inhibitors get inside the cell to kill the cancer, while monoclonal antibodies target specific receptors on lymphoma cells to initiate an immune response against the cancer.

Non-Hodgkin lymphoma originates in the cells [lymphocytes] of the immune system and results in tumors in the **lymph nodes** and the **spleen.**

CELL DIVISION INHIBITORS

MONOCLONAL ANTIBODIES

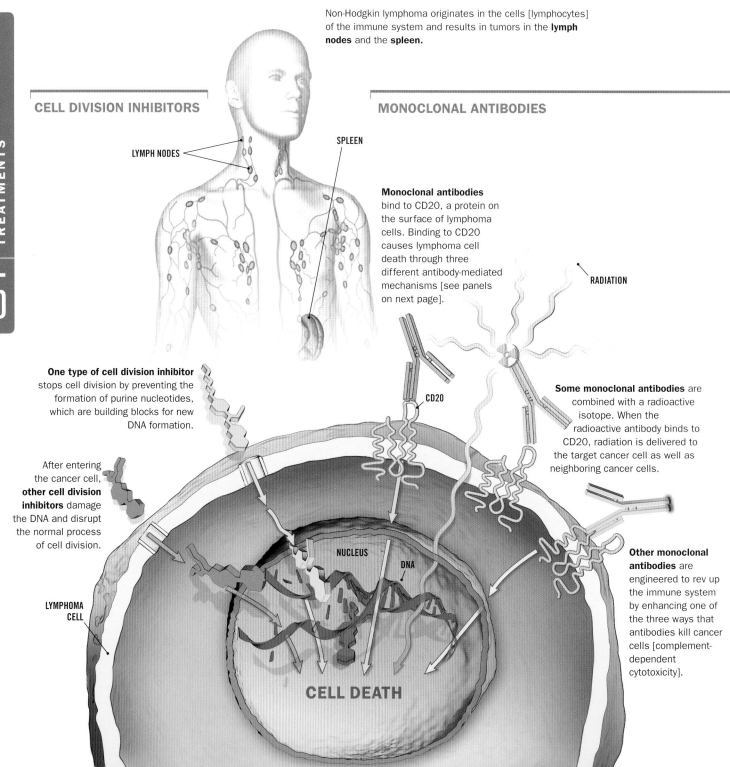

LYMPH NODES

SPLEEN

Monoclonal antibodies bind to CD20, a protein on the surface of lymphoma cells. Binding to CD20 causes lymphoma cell death through three different antibody-mediated mechanisms [see panels on next page].

RADIATION

One type of cell division inhibitor stops cell division by preventing the formation of purine nucleotides, which are building blocks for new DNA formation.

CD20

Some monoclonal antibodies are combined with a radioactive isotope. When the radioactive antibody binds to CD20, radiation is delivered to the target cancer cell as well as neighboring cancer cells.

After entering the cancer cell, **other cell division inhibitors** damage the DNA and disrupt the normal process of cell division.

NUCLEUS

DNA

Other monoclonal antibodies are engineered to rev up the immune system by enhancing one of the three ways that antibodies kill cancer cells [complement-dependent cytotoxicity].

LYMPHOMA CELL

CELL DEATH

The 3 Ways Monoclonal Antibodies Kill Cancer Cells

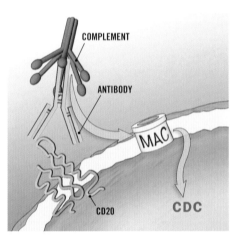

The Complement Cascade

A complement protein complex binds to the antibody and turns on the complement cascade. The end result is formation of the membrane attack complex [MAC], which creates a hole in the cell membrane that ultimately causes the cell to disintegrate. This process is known as complement-dependent cytotoxicity [CDC].

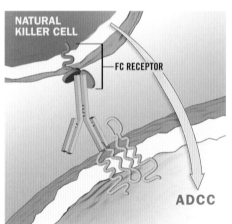

Natural Killer Cells

Antibodies that are attached to cancer cells attract natural killer [NK] cells, a type of white blood cell that circulates in the blood. A portion of the antibody called Fc binds to the Fc receptor on NK cells and initiates a process called antibody-dependent cellular cytotoxicity [ADCC] that destroys the cancer cell.

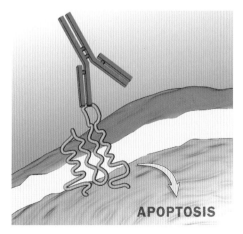

Cell Death From the Inside

Binding of antibodies to proteins on the surface of cancer cells can directly interfere with normal growth signals and activate a cell death pathway [apoptosis] inside the cell.

ILLUSTRATION BY ERIN MOORE
ORIGINALLY PUBLISHED IN "TRYING SOMETHING NEW," *CURE* SPRING 2009

Chronic Lymphocytic Leukemia Treatment

Depending on disease stage and the patient's prognostic factors, treatment may include observation, chemotherapy, radiation, surgery or stem cell transplantation.

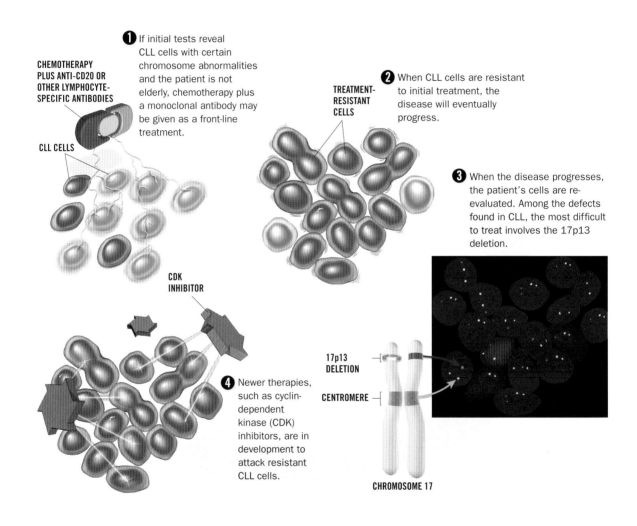

CHEMOTHERAPY PLUS ANTI-CD20 OR OTHER LYMPHOCYTE-SPECIFIC ANTIBODIES

CLL CELLS

1 If initial tests reveal CLL cells with certain chromosome abnormalities and the patient is not elderly, chemotherapy plus a monoclonal antibody may be given as a front-line treatment.

TREATMENT-RESISTANT CELLS

2 When CLL cells are resistant to initial treatment, the disease will eventually progress.

3 When the disease progresses, the patient's cells are re-evaluated. Among the defects found in CLL, the most difficult to treat involves the 17p13 deletion.

CDK INHIBITOR

4 Newer therapies, such as cyclin-dependent kinase (CDK) inhibitors, are in development to attack resistant CLL cells.

17p13 DELETION

CENTROMERE

CHROMOSOME 17

ILLUSTRATION BY ERIN MOORE
ORIGINALLY PUBLISHED IN "PROGRESS THAT'S WORTH THE WAIT," *CURE* SUMMER 2010

Vaccine Therapy

[Although a number of vaccines are available to prevent cancer, vaccines that treat existing cancer are either approved or currently being tested.]

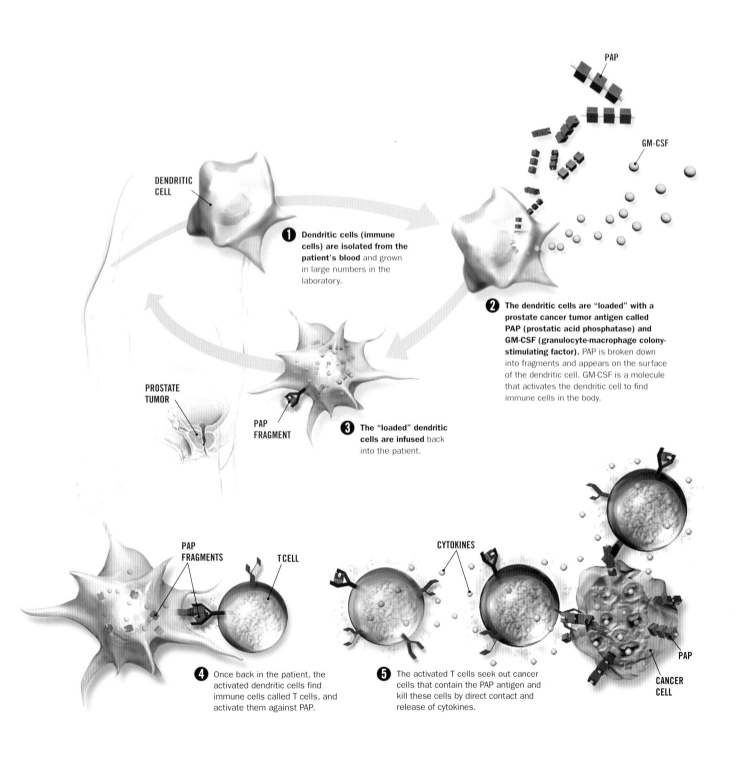

PAP

GM-CSF

DENDRITIC CELL

❶ **Dendritic cells (immune cells) are isolated from the patient's blood** and grown in large numbers in the laboratory.

❷ **The dendritic cells are "loaded" with a prostate cancer tumor antigen called PAP (prostatic acid phosphatase) and GM-CSF (granulocyte-macrophage colony-stimulating factor).** PAP is broken down into fragments and appears on the surface of the dendritic cell. GM-CSF is a molecule that activates the dendritic cell to find immune cells in the body.

PROSTATE TUMOR

PAP FRAGMENT

❸ **The "loaded" dendritic cells are infused** back into the patient.

PAP FRAGMENTS

T CELL

CYTOKINES

PAP

CANCER CELL

❹ Once back in the patient, the activated dendritic cells find immune cells called T cells, and activate them against PAP.

❺ The activated T cells seek out cancer cells that contain the PAP antigen and kill these cells by direct contact and release of cytokines.

ILLUSTRATION BY PAM CURRY
ORIGINALLY PUBLISHED IN "GETTING PERSONAL," *CURE* SPRING 2010

Targeting KRAS

Certain drugs target different pathways, depending on the tumor cell's biology.
Experimental drugs attack cancer by blocking alternate growth pathways.

NORMAL KRAS >

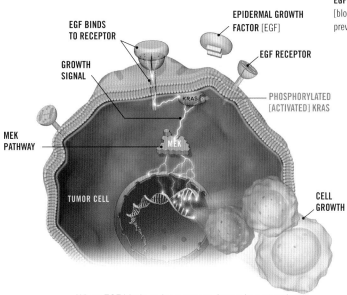

EPIDERMAL GROWTH FACTOR [EGF]

EGF BINDS TO RECEPTOR

GROWTH SIGNAL

EGF RECEPTOR

KRAS

PHOSPHORYLATED [ACTIVATED] KRAS

MEK PATHWAY

MEK

TUMOR CELL

CELL GROWTH

When EGF binds to its receptor, it sends a growth signal via the RAS pathway, **turning KRAS "on"** and transmitting a downstream signal **for the cancer cell to multiply.**

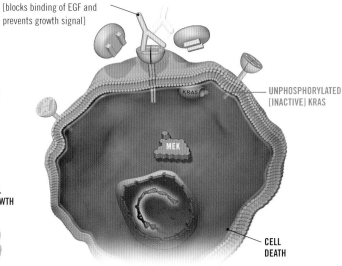

EGFR INHIBITOR
[blocks binding of EGF and prevents growth signal]

KRAS

UNPHOSPHORYLATED [INACTIVE] KRAS

MEK

CELL DEATH

If KRAS is normal, an **EGFR inhibitor** can successfully block the growth signal, **thus keeping KRAS turned "off" and causing the cancer cells to die.**

MUTATED KRAS >

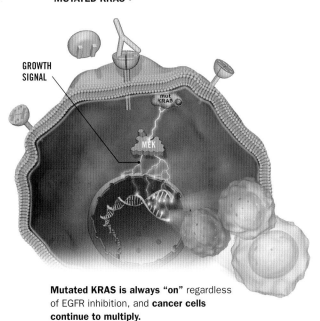

GROWTH SIGNAL

mut KRAS

MEK

Mutated KRAS is always "on" regardless of EGFR inhibition, and **cancer cells continue to multiply.**

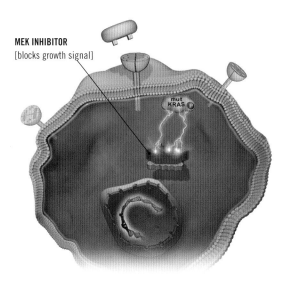

MEK INHIBITOR
[blocks growth signal]

mut KRAS

Drugs such as **MEK inhibitors** attempt to **bypass the RAS pathway and kill the cancer** by blocking the growth-signaling pathway further downstream from KRAS.

ILLUSTRATION BY ERIN MOORE
ORIGINALLY PUBLISHED IN "BITTERSWEET GENE," *CURE* WINTER 2008

Immunotherapies

[Immunotherapy breaks the immune system's tolerance of cancer cells through stimulation of key immune cells and proteins.]

NORMAL IMMUNE RESPONSE

Cells, such as antigen-presenting cells and lymphocytes [white blood cells], regulate the immune response when "foreign" pathogens are found. ›

INFECTED CELLS

FOREIGN PATHOGENS

CYTOTOXIC T CELLS

❸ Stimulatory cytokines activate cytotoxic T cells to attack infected cells.

CTLA-4 PROTEIN

B7

LYMPHOCYTE

ACTIVATED IMMUNE RESPONSE

ANTIGEN-PRESENTING CELL [APC]

STIMULATORY CYTOKINES

❷ APC signals the lymphocyte to release stimulatory cytokines.

❶ APC locates and absorbs foreign pathogens.

T CELLS

IMMUNOTHERAPY

Below are three ways to stimulate the body's natural immune response against cancer:

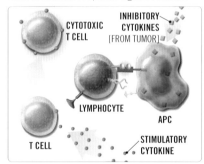

CYTOTOXIC T CELL

INHIBITORY CYTOKINES [FROM TUMOR]

LYMPHOCYTE

APC

T CELL

STIMULATORY CYTOKINE

Stimulatory cytokines: Cancer cells evade the body's natural immune response by releasing inhibitory cytokines that suppress the immune system. Stimulatory cytokines are used as therapy to override the inhibitory cytokines and activate cytotoxic T cells, which seek out and destroy the tumor.

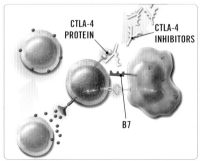

CTLA-4 PROTEIN

CTLA-4 INHIBITORS

B7

CTLA-4 Inhibitors: CTLA-4 is a protein that normally interacts with B7 on the APC to stop the immune response. CTLA-4 inhibitors are antibodies that block the binding of CTLA-4 to B7, causing the body's natural defenses to stay elevated and the immune system to continue attacking tumor cells.

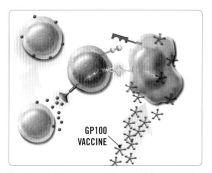

GP100 VACCINE

Vaccines: By incorporating gp100, a protein commonly found on melanoma cells, into the APC, the vaccine stimulates an immune response specifically against cancer cells that express gp100.

CTLA-4 Inhibitors

Although the immune system is primed to kill abnormal or "foreign" cells, it can be tricked into telling the body to turn off this response. CTLA-4 inhibitors interrupt that signal.

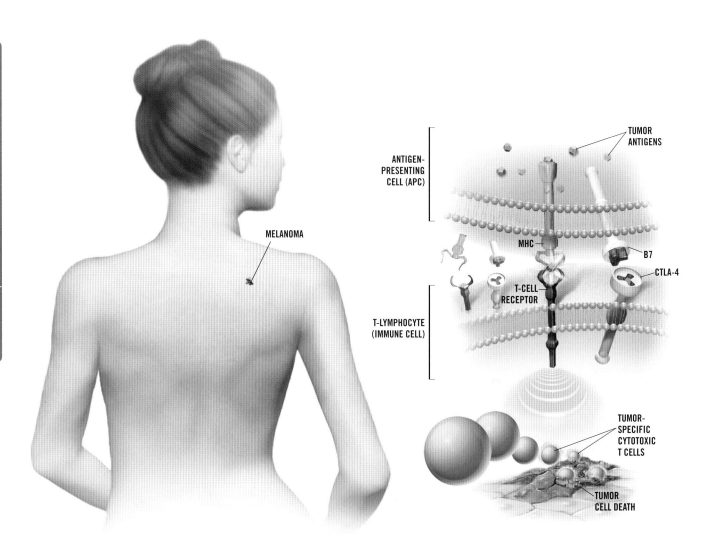

MELANOMA

TUMOR ANTIGENS

ANTIGEN-PRESENTING CELL (APC)

MHC

B7

CTLA-4

T-CELL RECEPTOR

T-LYMPHOCYTE (IMMUNE CELL)

TUMOR-SPECIFIC CYTOTOXIC T CELLS

TUMOR CELL DEATH

NORMAL IMMUNE RESPONSE › Certain immune cells, called antigen-presenting cells (APCs), will take "foreign" antigens, such as virus proteins or abnormal proteins made by cancer cells, and further process them via the major histocompatibility complex (MHC)–presenting molecule so they activate T cells. T cells, another immune cell type, have the ability to kill cells bearing foreign antigens.

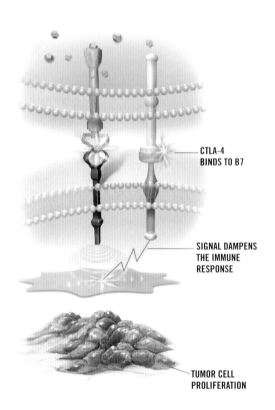

CTLA-4
BINDS TO B7

SIGNAL DAMPENS
THE IMMUNE
RESPONSE

TUMOR CELL
PROLIFERATION

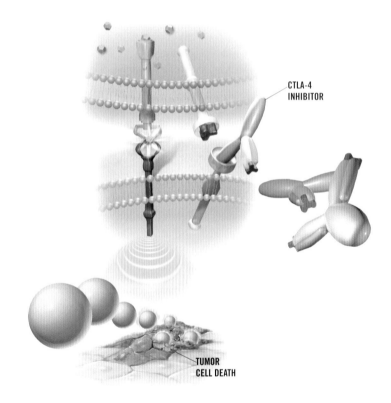

CTLA-4
INHIBITOR

TUMOR
CELL DEATH

IMMUNE RESPONSE DAMPENED › Once a T cell is activated, it triggers CTLA-4 proteins, which interact with the APC by binding to B7 proteins. When these proteins bind together, they send a "shut-off" signal to dampen the immune response, allowing cells to proliferate.

DAMPENING INTERRUPTED ›
By binding to the CTLA-4 protein, a CTLA-4 inhibitor interrupts the "shut-off" signal, enabling the immune system to attack the tumor cells.

ILLUSTRATION BY PAM CURRY
ORIGINALLY PUBLISHED IN "READY FOR TAKEOFF," *CURE* SUMMER 2011

BRAF Inhibitors

Uncontrolled cell growth can occur when a BRAF gene becomes mutated. BRAF inhibitors work to block that growth signal and can result in tumor death.

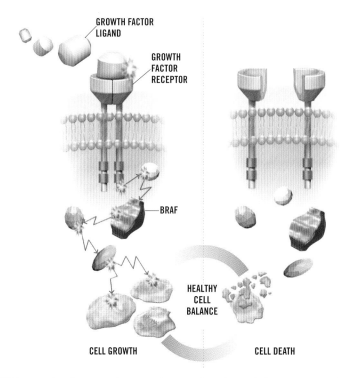

GROWTH FACTOR LIGAND

GROWTH FACTOR RECEPTOR

BRAF

HEALTHY CELL BALANCE

CELL GROWTH

CELL DEATH

CELL GROWTH is a regulated process. It commonly occurs through growth factor receptors that are activated by binding to growth factor ligands, setting off signals through intermediaries (including the BRAF protein) and leading to cell division. In the absence of growth factor ligand, healthy cells will not divide.

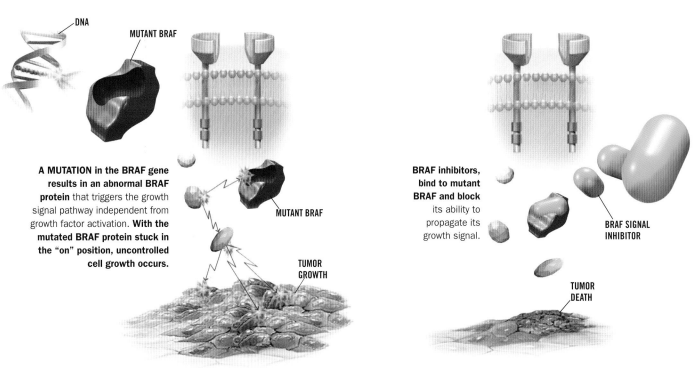

DNA

MUTANT BRAF

A MUTATION in the BRAF gene results in an abnormal BRAF protein that triggers the growth signal pathway independent from growth factor activation. **With the mutated BRAF protein stuck in the "on" position, uncontrolled cell growth occurs.**

MUTANT BRAF

TUMOR GROWTH

BRAF inhibitors, bind to mutant BRAF and block its ability to propagate its growth signal.

BRAF SIGNAL INHIBITOR

TUMOR DEATH

ILLUSTRATION BY PAM CURRY
ORIGINALLY PUBLISHED IN "READY FOR TAKEOFF," *CURE* SUMMER 2011

TREATMENTS

5

Angiogenesis Inhibitors

Angiogenesis involves development and growth of new blood vessels that feed a tumor, which produces vascular endothelial growth factor (VEGF) protein.

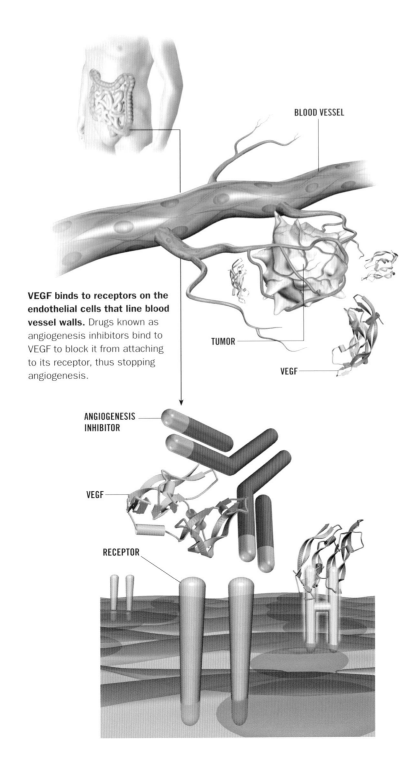

BLOOD VESSEL

VEGF binds to receptors on the endothelial cells that line blood vessel walls. Drugs known as angiogenesis inhibitors bind to VEGF to block it from attaching to its receptor, thus stopping angiogenesis.

TUMOR

VEGF

ANGIOGENESIS INHIBITOR

VEGF

RECEPTOR

Targeting HER2

[For about 20 percent of patients with advanced gastric cancer, tumors overproduce a receptor protein called HER2*.]

HER2, or human epidermal growth factor receptor 2, is found in normal amounts on the surface of some gastric cancer cells.

HER2 sometimes exists in abundance because there are extra copies of the HER2 gene [also known as HER2 gene amplification].

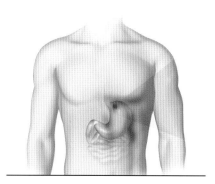

HER2

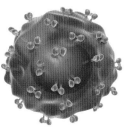

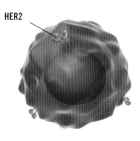

HER2 receptors transmit chemical signals that promote growth and survival of a cancer cell.

A drug known as a monoclonal antibody interferes with those signals and activates the immune system to promote destruction of the cell.

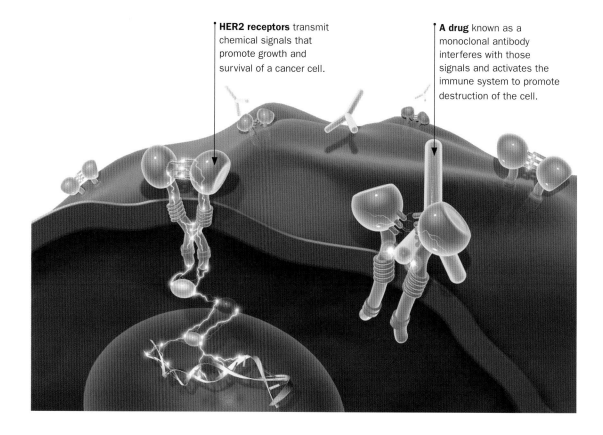

ILLUSTRATION BY ERIN MOORE
ORIGINALLY PUBLISHED IN "GUT REACTION," *CURE* WINTER 2009
*HER2 is also associated with breast cancer. For more information, see page 59.

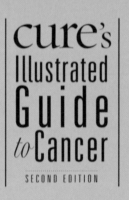

Chapter 6
Side Effects

CANCER TREATMENTS can cause side effects. Surgery may result in pain, bruising or infection. Chemotherapy can damage healthy tissue, triggering side effects such as neuropathy, mouth sores, nausea, vomiting, hair loss, low blood counts and weight changes. Radiation therapy can cause rash or hair loss in the treated area, fatigue and low blood cell counts. Most side effects fade after treatment ends and cells repair themselves. Other side effects persist for months or years after treatment. Long-term effects may start during treatment and endure for some time after treatment has ended. For example, neuropathy may start during chemotherapy but diminish or disappear as time passes. Late effects are side effects that appear months or years after treatment is completed. Examples of late effects from treatment are heart damage and secondary cancers.

Lymphedema

Surgery or radiation on the lymph nodes may result in lymphedema, a disruption in the flow of lymph fluid that causes swelling.

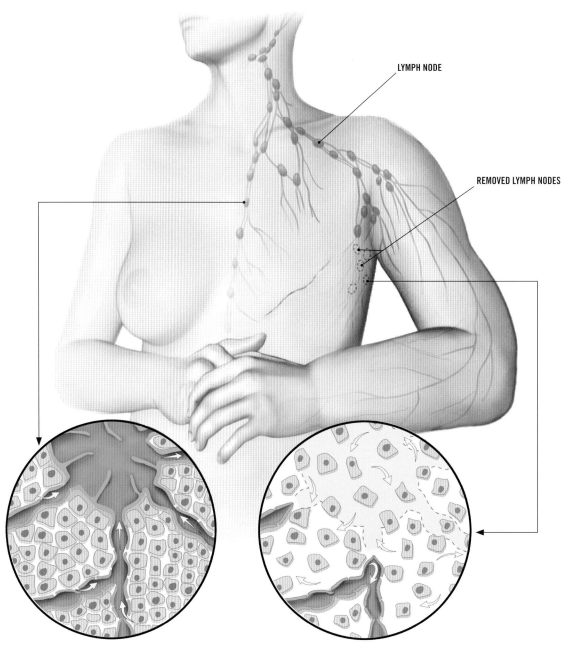

LYMPH NODE

REMOVED LYMPH NODES

Lymph nodes help maintain the body's fluid balance, filter out waste products and defend the body against threats, such as bacteria.

The normal flow of **lymphatic fluid** is disrupted when lymph nodes are removed or destroyed. Injury, infection or overuse can lead to a backup of fluid that causes swelling of the affected area.

ILLUSTRATION BY PAM CURRY
ORIGINALLY PUBLISHED IN *CURE'S ILLUSTRATED GUIDE TO CANCER*, 2010

Heart Damage

Some cancer treatments can damage the heart in different locations and in a variety of ways.

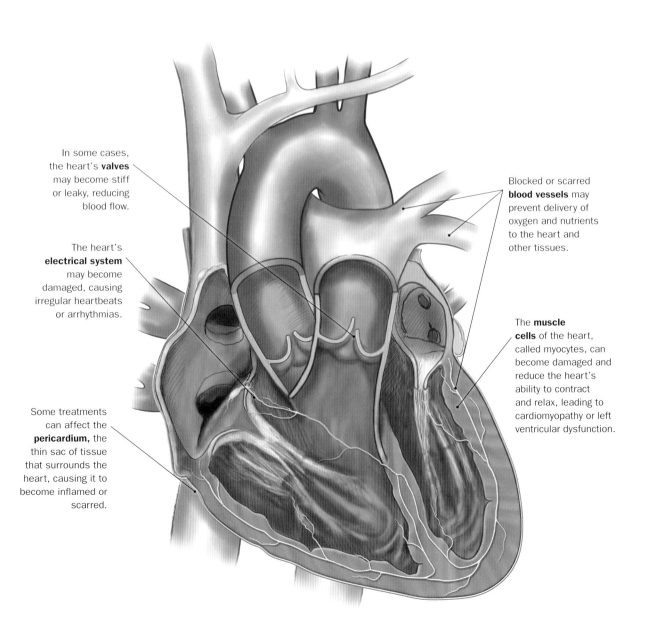

In some cases, the heart's **valves** may become stiff or leaky, reducing blood flow.

The heart's **electrical system** may become damaged, causing irregular heartbeats or arrhythmias.

Some treatments can affect the **pericardium,** the thin sac of tissue that surrounds the heart, causing it to become inflamed or scarred.

Blocked or scarred **blood vessels** may prevent delivery of oxygen and nutrients to the heart and other tissues.

The **muscle cells** of the heart, called myocytes, can become damaged and reduce the heart's ability to contract and relax, leading to cardiomyopathy or left ventricular dysfunction.

ILLUSTRATION BY ERIN MOORE
ORIGINALLY PUBLISHED IN "HAZARDOUS TO YOUR HEART," *CURE* SPRING 2007

MRSA Infection

MRSA is an antibiotic-resistant staph infection that can infect several areas of the body and cause serious illness.

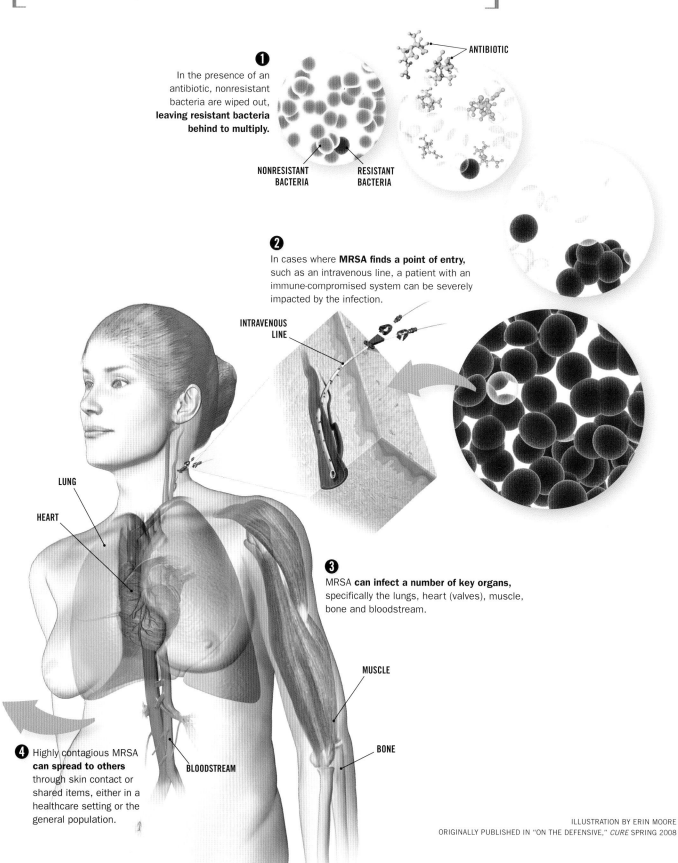

❶ In the presence of an antibiotic, nonresistant bacteria are wiped out, **leaving resistant bacteria behind to multiply.**

ANTIBIOTIC

NONRESISTANT BACTERIA

RESISTANT BACTERIA

❷ In cases where **MRSA finds a point of entry,** such as an intravenous line, a patient with an immune-compromised system can be severely impacted by the infection.

INTRAVENOUS LINE

LUNG

HEART

❸ MRSA **can infect a number of key organs,** specifically the lungs, heart (valves), muscle, bone and bloodstream.

MUSCLE

BONE

❹ Highly contagious MRSA **can spread to others** through skin contact or shared items, either in a healthcare setting or the general population.

BLOODSTREAM

ILLUSTRATION BY ERIN MOORE
ORIGINALLY PUBLISHED IN "ON THE DEFENSIVE," *CURE* SPRING 2008

Bone Loss

[Some treatments can cause bone tissue to break down, resulting in bones becoming weak and fragile. However, patients can take drugs to help prevent bone loss.]

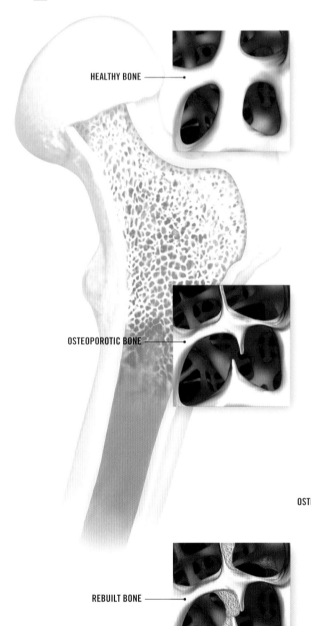

HEALTHY BONE

OSTEOPOROTIC BONE

REBUILT BONE

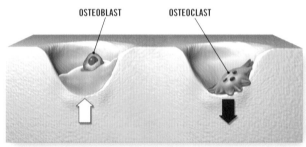

OSTEOBLAST   OSTEOCLAST

NORMAL BONE [HEALTHY BALANCE] › In normal bone, a delicate balance exists between cells that build up bone tissue, called osteoblasts, and cells that dissolve bone tissue (break it down), called osteoclasts. Estrogen plays a key role in maintaining this healthy balance and preserving bone density.

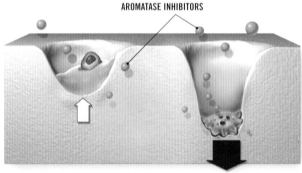

AROMATASE INHIBITORS

BONE LOSS [UNHEALTHY BALANCE] › Aromatase inhibitors treat breast cancer by inhibiting estrogen production, which, in turn, alters the amount of hormone that reaches bone cells. Without estrogen, bone loss outpaces bone deposition, making the bone more porous and susceptible to fracture.

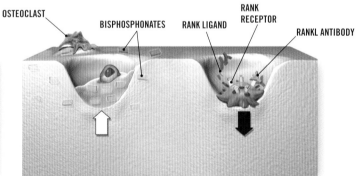

OSTEOCLAST   BISPHOSPHONATES   RANK LIGAND   RANK RECEPTOR   RANKL ANTIBODY

PREVENTING BONE LOSS ›

Bisphosphonates inhibit the activity of osteoclasts, while at the same time increase osteoblast activity by protecting the bone-building cells from dying. Although bisphosphonates also increase bone mineral density by incorporating themselves into the bone matrix, the quality of the bone may remain low.

RANK ligand (RANKL), a protein that tells the body to remove bone, is an important component of the normal bone matrix. Typically, RANKL activates osteoclasts by binding to the RANK receptor. Antibodies that bind RANKL can prevent this activation process.

ILLUSTRATION BY ERIN MOORE
ORIGINALLY PUBLISHED IN "GOOD TO THE BONE," *CURE* WINTER 2007

Pain

[Pain can be caused by cancer or its treatment but can often be relieved with an array of treatment strategies.]

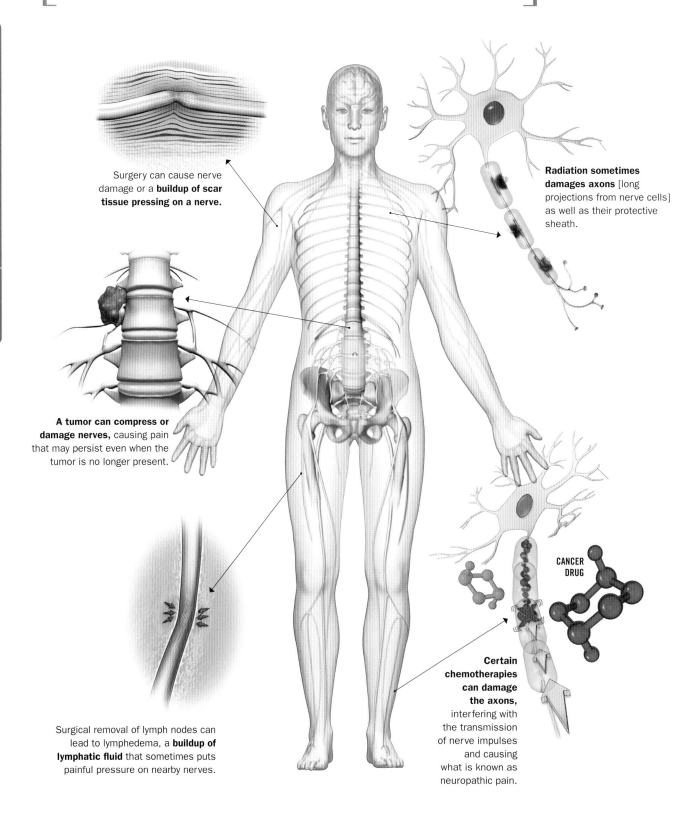

Surgery can cause nerve damage or a **buildup of scar tissue pressing on a nerve.**

Radiation sometimes damages axons [long projections from nerve cells] as well as their protective sheath.

A tumor can compress or damage nerves, causing pain that may persist even when the tumor is no longer present.

CANCER DRUG

Surgical removal of lymph nodes can lead to lymphedema, a **buildup of lymphatic fluid** that sometimes puts painful pressure on nearby nerves.

Certain chemotherapies can damage the axons, interfering with the transmission of nerve impulses and causing what is known as neuropathic pain.

ILLUSTRATION BY ERIN MOORE
ORIGINALLY PUBLISHED IN "HELP FOR WHERE IT HURTS," *HEAL* FALL 2007

Hair Loss

Hair loss is a common side effect that can result from radiation to a treated area or from some chemotherapies.

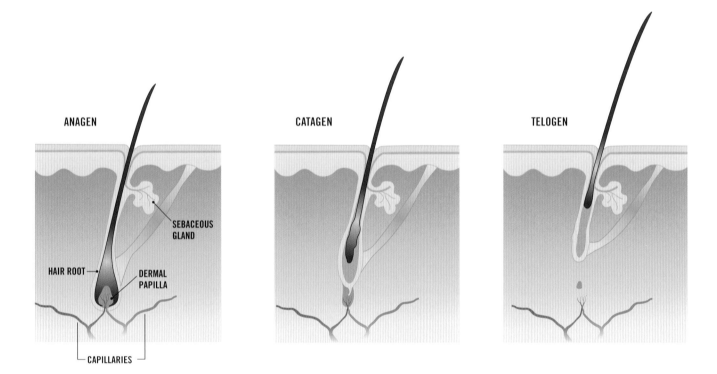

ANAGEN

SEBACEOUS GLAND

HAIR ROOT

DERMAL PAPILLA

CAPILLARIES

CATAGEN

TELOGEN

All hair follicles go through a cycle of growth (anagen), a transitional phase (catagen) and a terminal phase (telogen) when the older hair falls out and a new cycle of hair growth begins. Anagen is the longest phase, with up to 90 percent of follicles in that phase at any given time. The catagen phase is a transitional time when cell division slows. The telogen phase, the resting phase, is the point of hair loss. Chemotherapy affects the rapidly dividing cells in the bulb surrounding the dermal papilla, which is at the base of the hair follicle, causing hair loss. Patients who receive radiation to parts of the body where there is hair growth may lose hair in that area. Most patients will have their hair grow back once chemotherapy or radiation is completed.

ILLUSTRATION BY ERIN MOORE
ORIGINALLY PUBLISHED IN *CURE'S ILLUSTRATED GUIDE TO CANCER*, 2010

Nausea and Vomiting

Many antinausea drugs, called antiemetics, help patients with the nausea and vomiting that can accompany some treatments.

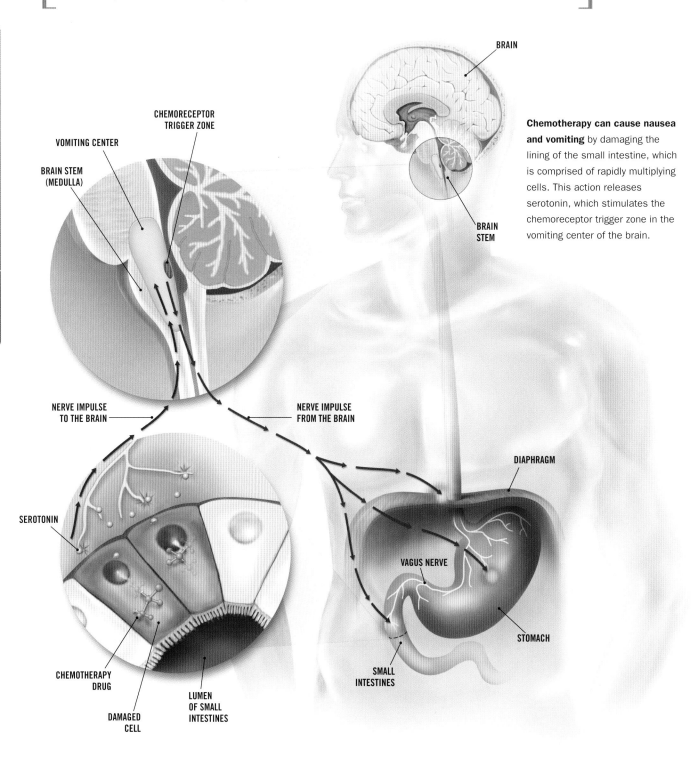

BRAIN

Chemotherapy can cause nausea and vomiting by damaging the lining of the small intestine, which is comprised of rapidly multiplying cells. This action releases serotonin, which stimulates the chemoreceptor trigger zone in the vomiting center of the brain.

BRAIN STEM

CHEMORECEPTOR TRIGGER ZONE

VOMITING CENTER

BRAIN STEM (MEDULLA)

NERVE IMPULSE TO THE BRAIN

NERVE IMPULSE FROM THE BRAIN

DIAPHRAGM

SEROTONIN

VAGUS NERVE

CHEMOTHERAPY DRUG

DAMAGED CELL

LUMEN OF SMALL INTESTINES

SMALL INTESTINES

STOMACH

ILLUSTRATION BY PAM CURRY
ORIGINALLY PUBLISHED IN *CURE'S ILLUSTRATED GUIDE TO CANCER*, 2010

Neutropenia

Chemotherapy or radiation can inhibit the production of white blood cells, called neutrophils, which can result in neutropenia, making a patient more prone to infection.

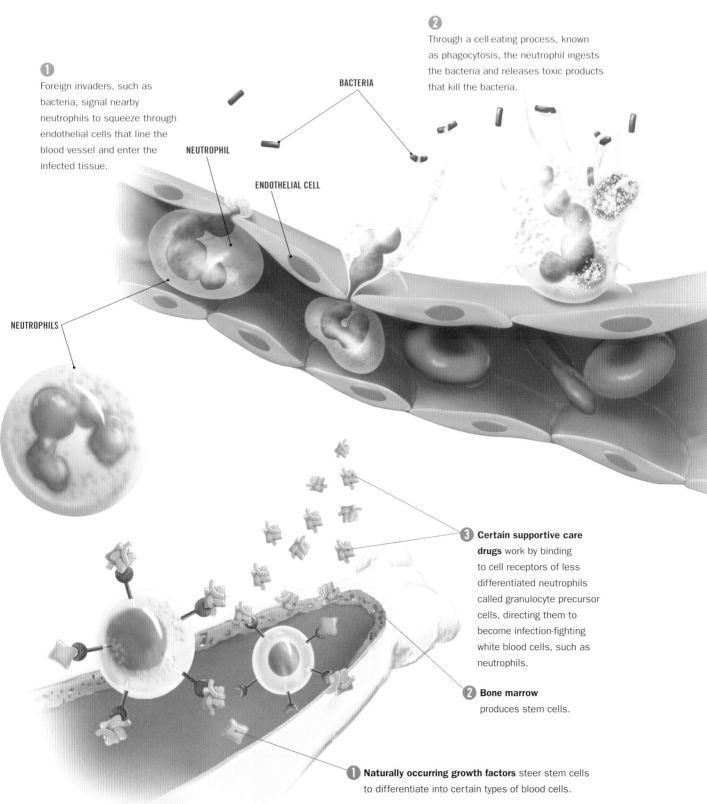

1 Foreign invaders, such as bacteria, signal nearby neutrophils to squeeze through endothelial cells that line the blood vessel and enter the infected tissue.

2 Through a cell-eating process, known as phagocytosis, the neutrophil ingests the bacteria and releases toxic products that kill the bacteria.

BACTERIA

NEUTROPHIL

ENDOTHELIAL CELL

NEUTROPHILS

3 **Certain supportive care drugs** work by binding to cell receptors of less differentiated neutrophils called granulocyte precursor cells, directing them to become infection-fighting white blood cells, such as neutrophils.

2 **Bone marrow** produces stem cells.

1 **Naturally occurring growth factors** steer stem cells to differentiate into certain types of blood cells.

ILLUSTRATION BY PAM CURRY
ORIGINALLY PUBLISHED IN "RUNNING ON EMPTY," *CURE* SUMMER 2006

Peripheral Neuropathy

Peripheral neuropathy results from damage to the nervous system and may cause pain, numbness, tingling or loss of sensation.

Neuropathy can be caused by radiation to the nerves or by a tumor close to the nerves. However, more commonly, neuropathy is caused by certain chemotherapies that damage the nerves or their environment. Nerves run up and down the body from the spine to the toes. Some patients describe the loss of sensations caused by neuropathy as similar to the feeling of wearing a stocking or glove.

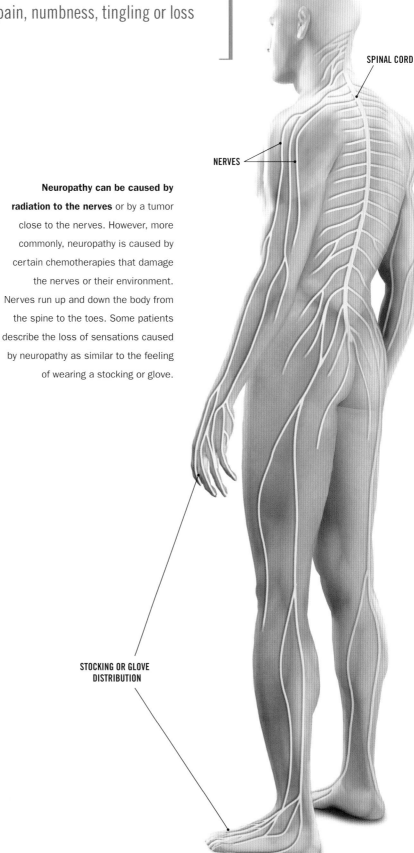

SPINAL CORD

NERVES

STOCKING OR GLOVE DISTRIBUTION

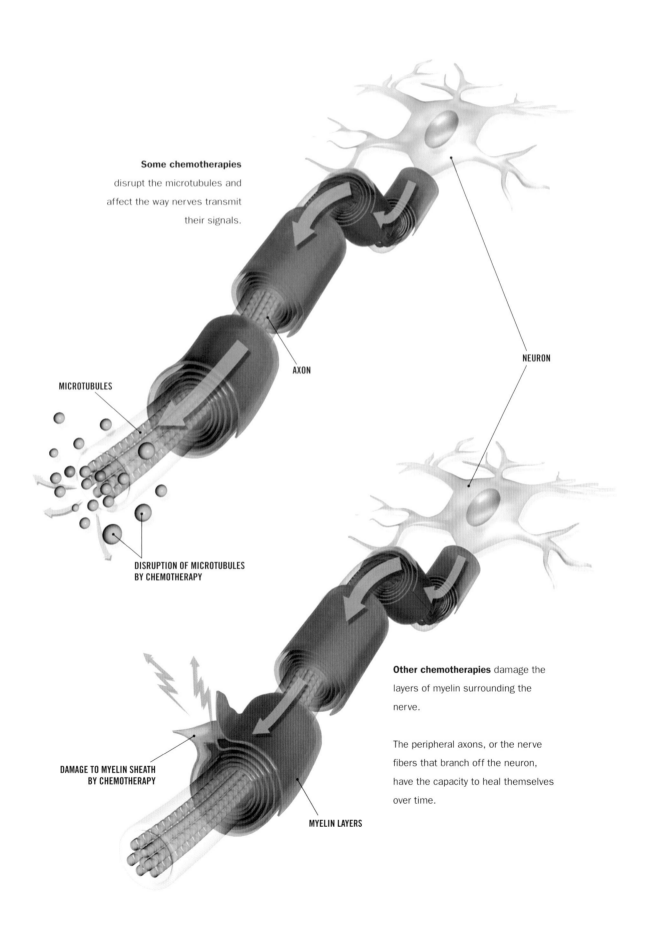

Some chemotherapies disrupt the microtubules and affect the way nerves transmit their signals.

NEURON

MICROTUBULES

AXON

DISRUPTION OF MICROTUBULES BY CHEMOTHERAPY

Other chemotherapies damage the layers of myelin surrounding the nerve.

The peripheral axons, or the nerve fibers that branch off the neuron, have the capacity to heal themselves over time.

DAMAGE TO MYELIN SHEATH BY CHEMOTHERAPY

MYELIN LAYERS

ILLUSTRATION BY PAM CURRY & ERIN MOORE
ORIGINALLY PUBLISHED IN *CURE'S ILLUSTRATED GUIDE TO CANCER*, 2010

Complications of the Mouth and Throat

Most cancers of the head and neck are treated with surgery, radiation, chemotherapy and targeted drug therapy, either alone or in combination, all of which may cause side effects.

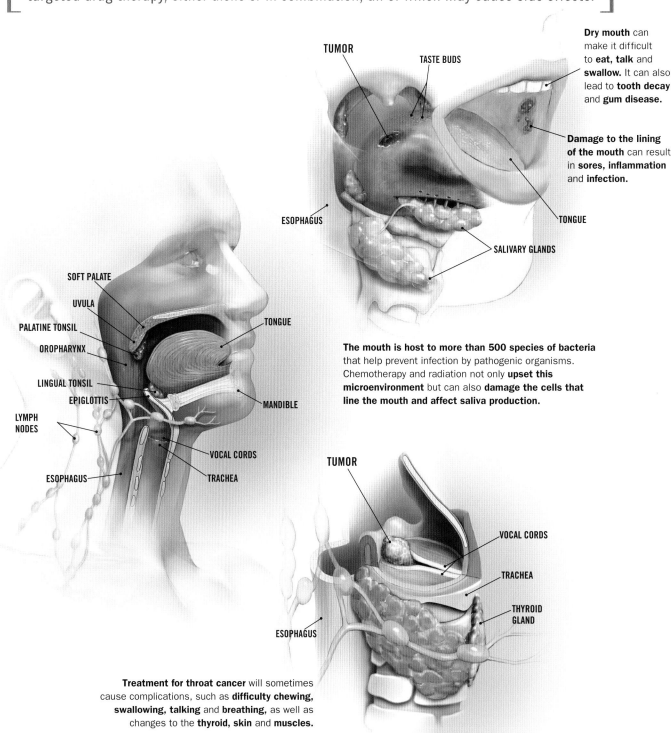

TUMOR

TASTE BUDS

Dry mouth can make it difficult to **eat, talk** and **swallow.** It can also lead to **tooth decay** and **gum disease.**

Damage to the lining of the mouth can result in **sores, inflammation** and **infection.**

ESOPHAGUS

TONGUE

SALIVARY GLANDS

SOFT PALATE

UVULA

PALATINE TONSIL

OROPHARYNX

LINGUAL TONSIL

EPIGLOTTIS

LYMPH NODES

ESOPHAGUS

TONGUE

MANDIBLE

VOCAL CORDS

TRACHEA

The mouth is host to more than 500 species of bacteria that help prevent infection by pathogenic organisms. Chemotherapy and radiation not only **upset this microenvironment** but can also **damage the cells that line the mouth and affect saliva production.**

TUMOR

VOCAL CORDS

TRACHEA

THYROID GLAND

ESOPHAGUS

Treatment for throat cancer will sometimes cause complications, such as **difficulty chewing, swallowing, talking** and **breathing,** as well as changes to the **thyroid, skin** and **muscles.**

ILLUSTRATION BY PAM CURRY
ORIGINALLY PUBLISHED IN "FACING THE FACTS," *CURE* SUMMER 2012

Blood Clots

Some cancer survivors find that radiation treatments can cause problems down the road.

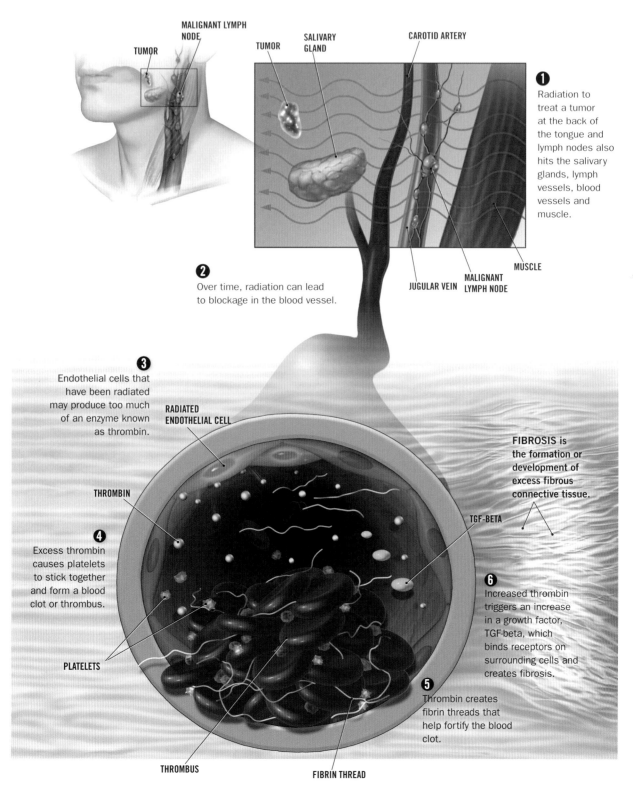

MALIGNANT LYMPH NODE

TUMOR

TUMOR

SALIVARY GLAND

CAROTID ARTERY

❶ Radiation to treat a tumor at the back of the tongue and lymph nodes also hits the salivary glands, lymph vessels, blood vessels and muscle.

MUSCLE

JUGULAR VEIN

MALIGNANT LYMPH NODE

❷ Over time, radiation can lead to blockage in the blood vessel.

❸ Endothelial cells that have been radiated may produce too much of an enzyme known as thrombin.

RADIATED ENDOTHELIAL CELL

THROMBIN

FIBROSIS is the formation or development of excess fibrous connective tissue.

TGF-BETA

❹ Excess thrombin causes platelets to stick together and form a blood clot or thrombus.

PLATELETS

❻ Increased thrombin triggers an increase in a growth factor, TGF-beta, which binds receptors on surrounding cells and creates fibrosis.

❺ Thrombin creates fibrin threads that help fortify the blood clot.

THROMBUS

FIBRIN THREAD

ILLUSTRATION BY ERIN MOORE
ORIGINALLY PUBLISHED IN "THE COST OF LIVING," *CURE* WINTER 2010

Weight Loss or Gain

Signals to the brain from the stomach initiate hunger, while serotonin released from the brain signals a feeling of fullness. Certain drugs effect weight loss or gain.

SIDE EFFECTS

6

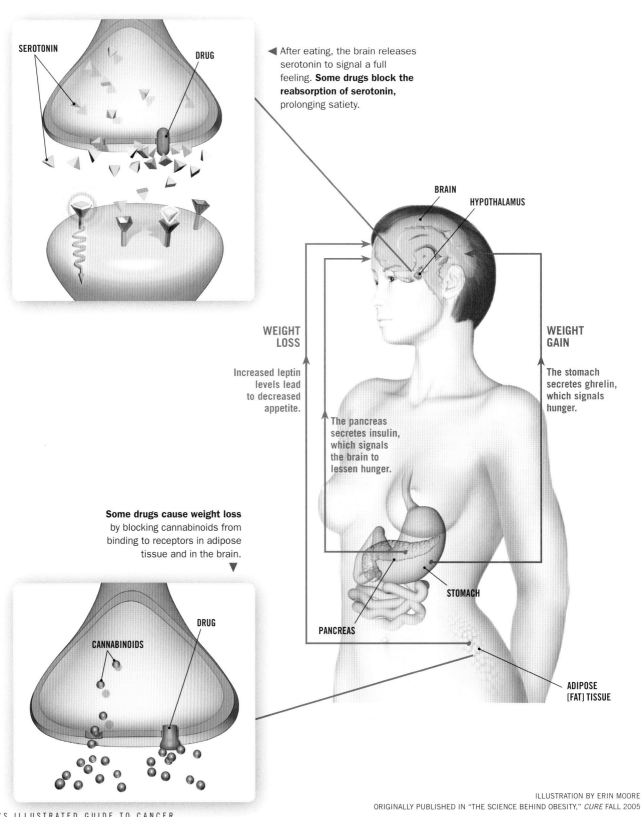

SEROTONIN

DRUG

◄ After eating, the brain releases serotonin to signal a full feeling. **Some drugs block the reabsorption of serotonin,** prolonging satiety.

BRAIN

HYPOTHALAMUS

WEIGHT LOSS

Increased leptin levels lead to decreased appetite.

WEIGHT GAIN

The stomach secretes ghrelin, which signals hunger.

The pancreas secretes insulin, which signals the brain to lessen hunger.

Some drugs cause weight loss by blocking cannabinoids from binding to receptors in adipose tissue and in the brain.
▼

STOMACH

CANNABINOIDS

DRUG

PANCREAS

ADIPOSE [FAT] TISSUE

ILLUSTRATION BY ERIN MOORE
ORIGINALLY PUBLISHED IN "THE SCIENCE BEHIND OBESITY," *CURE* FALL 2005

The Language of Cancer

Adenocarcinoma › Cancer that starts in the glandular tissue, such as in the ducts or lobules of the breast.

Angiogenesis › The formation of new blood vessels. Some cancer treatments work by blocking angiogenesis, thus preventing blood from reaching the tumor.

Antigen › A substance that causes the body's immune system to respond. This response often involves making antibodies. For example, the immune system's response to antigens that are part of bacteria and viruses helps people resist infections. Cancer cells have certain antigens that can be found by lab tests. They are important in cancer diagnosis and in watching response to treatment. Other cancer cell antigens play a role in immune reactions that may help the body's resistance against cancer.

Biopsy › The removal of a sample of tissue to see whether cancer cells are present. There are several different kinds of biopsies. In some, a very thin needle is used to draw fluid and cells from a lump. In a core biopsy, a larger needle is used to remove more tissue.

Brachytherapy › Internal radiation treatment given by placing radioactive material directly into the tumor or close to it.

Cancer › Develops when cells with damaged DNA begin to grow out of control.

Carcinoma › A malignant tumor that begins in the lining layer (epithelial cells) of organs. The most frequent cancers of this type in the U.S. are lung, breast, colon and prostate.

Chemotherapy › Systemic treatment with drugs to inhibit cancer cell division. Chemotherapy is often used with surgery or radiation to treat cancer when the cancer has spread, when it has come back (recurred) or when there is a strong chance it could recur.

Clinical trials › Research studies that test new drugs or treatments and compare them with current standard treatments. Before a new treatment is used on people, it is studied in the lab. If lab studies suggest the treatment works, it is tested for patients. These human studies are called clinical trials.

Cytokine › A product of cells of the immune system that may stimulate immunity and cause the regression of some cancers.

Cytotoxic › Toxic to cells; cell-killing.

DNA (deoxyribonucleic acid) › The genetic "blueprint" found in the nucleus of each cell. DNA holds genetic information on cell growth, division and function.

Enzyme › A protein that increases the rate of chemical reactions in living cells.

Estrogen › A female sex hormone produced primarily by the ovaries and in smaller amounts by the adrenal cortex. In breast cancer, estrogen may promote the growth of cancer cells.

Gene › A segment of DNA that contains information on hereditary characteristics, such as hair color, eye color and height, as well as susceptibility to certain diseases.

Genetic testing › Tests performed to determine whether a person has certain gene changes known to increase cancer risk. Such testing is recommended for those with specific types of family history. Genetic counseling should be part of the process.

Grade › Reflects how abnormal the cancer looks under the microscope. There are several grading systems for different types of cancer. Each grading system divides cancer into those with the greatest abnormality, the least abnormality and those in between. Cancers with more abnormal-appearing cells tend to grow and spread more quickly and have a worse prognosis.

Graft-versus-host disease › A condition that results when the immune cells of a transplantation (usually of stem cells) from a donor attack the tissues of the person receiving the transplant.

Growth factors › A naturally occurring protein that causes cells to grow and divide. Too much growth factor production by some cancer cells helps them grow quickly. Other growth factors help normal cells recover from side effects of chemotherapy.

Hormonal therapy › Treatment with drugs that interfere with hormone production or hormone action, or the surgical removal of hormone-producing glands. Hormonal therapy may kill cancer cells or slow their growth.

Immunotherapy › Treatments that promote or support the body's immune system response to a disease such as cancer.

Leukemia › Cancer of the blood or blood-forming organs. People with leukemia often have a noticeable increase in white blood cells (leukocytes).

Localized (or local) cancer › A cancer that is confined to the organ where it started; that is, it has not spread to distant parts of the body.

Lymph nodes › Small bean-shaped collections of immune system tissue, such as lymphocytes, found along lymphatic vessels. They remove cell waste, germs and other harmful substances from the lymph. They help fight infections and also have a role in fighting cancer, although cancers sometimes spread through the lymph system.

Lymphoma › A cancer of the lymphatic system, a network of thin vessels and nodes throughout the body. Lymphoma involves a type of white blood cells called lymphocytes. The two main types of lymphoma are Hodgkin and non-Hodgkin.

Malignant › A mass of cells that may invade nearby tissues or spread (metastasize) to distant areas of the body.

Metastasis › Cancer cells that have spread to one or more sites elsewhere in the body, often by way of the lymph system or bloodstream. Regional metastasis is cancer that has spread to the lymph nodes, tissues or organs close to the primary site. Distant metastasis is cancer that has spread to organs or tissues that are farther away (such as when prostate cancer spreads to the bones, lungs or liver).

Monoclonal antibodies › Antibodies made in the lab to lock onto specific antigens.

Mutation › A change in the DNA of a cell. Cancer is thought to be due to mutations that damage a cell's DNA. Most mutations happen after the person is born.

Pathologist › A doctor who specializes in diagnosis and classification of diseases by lab tests such as examining cells under a microscope. The pathologist determines the specifics of a diagnosis.

Radiation therapy › Treatment with high-energy rays (such as X-rays) to kill or shrink cancer cells. The radiation may come from outside of the body (external radiation) or from radioactive materials placed directly in the tumor (brachytherapy or internal radiation).

Recurrence › The return of cancer after treatment. Local recurrence means that the cancer has come back in the same location as the original cancer. Regional recurrence means that the cancer has come back after treatment in the lymph nodes near the primary site. Distant recurrence is when cancer metastasizes after treatment to distant organs or tissues (such as the lungs, liver, bone marrow or brain).

Remission › Complete or partial disappearance of the signs and symptoms of cancer in response to treatment. A remission may not be a cure.

Sarcoma › A malignant tumor growing from connective tissues, such as cartilage, fat, muscle or bone.

Side effects › Unwanted effects of treatment that can include hair loss, anemia (low red blood cell count), fatigue, thrombocytopenia (low platelet count) and neuropathy (nerve damage).

Stage › Designation that indicates if and how far the cancer has spread. There is more than one system for staging different types of cancer. The most commonly used is the TNM staging system, which gives three key pieces of information: T stands for tumor (its size and how far it has spread to nearby tissues); N describes whether the cancer has spread to lymph nodes; M stands for spread (metastasis) to distant organs. All of this information is combined to assign the stage of the cancer. After stage 0 (which is carcinoma in situ or cancer that has not grown beyond the lining layer of cells), stages are labeled using numbers 1 through 4. The smaller the number, the less the cancer has spread. A higher number means a more advanced disease.

Stem cell transplantation › A procedure used to restock stem cells when they have been destroyed by chemotherapy, radiation or disease. Stem cells may be the patient's own (autologous) or may come from someone else (allogeneic). Bone marrow transplantations were the first method for replacing stem cells.

Targeted therapy › Treatment to attack the part of cancer cells that make them different from normal cells. Targeted agents tend to have different side effects than conventional chemotherapy drugs.

Adapted with permission of the American Cancer Society (cancer.org).

Index

At Genentech BioOncology, we're leading the fight against cancer with innovative science and fundamentally transforming the way cancer is treated. Our commitment to this goal has enabled us to make significant contributions to the understanding of cancer and to translate this understanding into targeted, biologic-based therapies.

BIO⊗NCOLOGY™

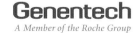
Genentech
A Member of the Roche Group